'This is a timely book on a vitally important subject. Raoul Goldberg focuses our attention on the battle for consciousness required to address our multiple mind-numbing and life-draining addictions.'

DR ROSY DANIEL, DIRECTOR OF THE BRITISH COLLEGE
OF INTEGRATIVE MEDICINE

—

'Dr Goldberg is the one of the most creative, original thinkers and researchers in the field of Integrative Medicine I have ever met, and a great contributor to the huge task of humanising medicine. He is a leading practitioner in the new field of Medical Psychophonetics, and his unique insight into the welfare of growing children, and into the formation and the possible healing of addiction in childhood, is a combination of years of devotional medical work with children with the depth of a great human soul.'

YEHUDA TAGAR, FOUNDER OF PSYCHOPHONETICS,
DIRECTOR OF PERSEPHONE INSTITUTE OF
PSYCHOPHONETICS AND OF MICHAELI LEADERSHIP
INSTITUTE (SOUTH AFRICA)

—

'A challenging yet hopeful book which tackles the core of a critical issue.'

PETER POWIS, CLINICAL PSYCHOLOGIST/
PSYCHOTHERAPIST, SYRINGA HEALTH CENTRE,
SOUTH AFRICA

—

About the Author

Dr Raoul Goldberg has practised Integrative Medicine for thirty-five years in Switzerland, Germany and the majority of his career in his homeland, South Africa. His work includes managing an Integrative Health Clinic and practising as a clinical doctor and counsellor, school doctor, international lecturer and child health researcher. He is the author of *Awakening to Child Health* (Hawthorn Press, UK) and many other publications on Integrative Medicine and Child Health.

Dr Goldberg has developed a unique brand of integrative medicine which combines anthroposophical medicine, homeopathy, functional medicine, nutritional medicine, psychophonetic counselling and life coaching, where the patient or client is an active partner in the diagnostic and therapeutic programme. He calls this *Participatory Medicine*.

In his consulting, writing and speaking he uses a technique of awakening and empowering deep inner healing experience which he calls *Awakening to Deep Experience*. This methodology brings together Psychophonetics, psychosophy, Goetheanistic science, drama and movement therapy, therapeutic arts and crafts, pedagogical science and other modalities. It is aimed at challenging and training people to sharpen their natural perceptive, cognitive, feeling and expressive capacities to gain deeper insight and empathy for their own wellbeing, for that of others and for the wellbeing of the world we live in.

Addictive Behaviour in Children and Young Adults

The Struggle For Freedom

RAOUL GOLDBERG MD

Floris Books

Published by Floris Books in 2012
© 2012 Raoul Goldberg MD

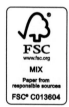

British Library CIP Data available
ISBN 987-086315-873-5
Printed in Great Britain
by CPI Group (UK) Ltd, Croydon

Contents

Acknowledgments

The writing of this book was made possible through two principal elements.

One was the emergence, over many years, of a methodology which I have employed throughout this work. This methodology came together through the meeting of various sources of inspiration and learning that I was privileged over three decades to experience, absorb and digest. I am indebted to the teachers of each of these fields of enquiry and wish to acknowledge chronologically each contribution that allowed this methodology to come to fruition: Rudolf Steiner, one of the foremost researchers and educators of our times, opened up for me a new paradigm of knowledge and experience, as well as an approach to experiencing these new frontiers, validating what was living as truth within me. Medical colleagues, who over my years of study, have enriched my medical insights and practice include Drs Rita Leroi, Herbert Sieweke, Otto Wolff, Bernard Lievegoed, Lothar Vogel, Rudolf Treichler, Klaus Wilde and Michaela Glöckler. Jochen Bockemühl, Goethean scientist, presented me with an approach to observing nature in a multifaceted way, using different modes of experience and expanding perceptive awareness. Yehuda Tagar, the founder of psychophonetics, introduced me to the dramatic inner life of the psyche and enabled me to research the vast expanse and resources of the human psyche by providing the tools to explore and manage these hidden realities.

The other element which provided the raw material for this book were the many clients, especially the children and adolescents, who allowed me into their inner space and gave me the privilege to accompany them into their world of addictive behaviour. They have validated my own experience of needs, dependency and gratification and have allowed me to present an approach which I believe is applicable and effective for most addictive young people. I also wish to express my gratitude to those parents who allowed me to make use of the case stories of their children.

There are a number of other people who contributed to the fullness and completion of this work and to whom I wish to acknowledge my gratitude: Dana Smirin, my partner, who gave me immense moral support and helped edit the book through her fine critique and objectivity; Peter Powis, clinical psychologist and addiction specialist, who conducted a professional edit of the book; Christian Maclean and Katy Lockwood-Holmes, who by publishing this work, put their trust in me to create a work they believe has relevance for the youth of today; Christopher Moore who took on the task of editing this work; Angela MacPherson, the artist who has captured so sensitively, pictures from the inner world of the psyche that represent some of the addictive agencies; Dalene Totten, editor of the *South African Journal of Natural Medicine,* who published seven articles on Addictive Behaviour in Children and Adolescents, forming the core content of this book.

Finally I wish to acknowledge the inexhaustible and indefatigable free spirit living within each and every human being that inspires and empowers the human psyche to strive to be free of the heavy chains of dependency and to open up space for the free will of the spirit to express itself.

Raoul Goldberg

Preface

In this, his second book, Raoul Goldberg has turned his attention to one of the most burning problems of our time: the issue of pervasive addiction and the difficult question of how to prevent it. On the one hand this has resulted in a book based on his rich experience as a family doctor and his advisory work in the field of education. On the other it addresses questions of how to find meaning in, and come to terms with, addiction, especially when the craving is attached to destructive inclinations such as sexual perversions and abuse.

Particularly interesting and illuminating is the book's inclusion of the results of spiritual research by Rudolf Steiner, the life reformer, cultural philosopher and visionary for the twenty-first century whose one hundred and fiftieth anniversary was celebrated worldwide in 2011. As a paediatrician and colleague from Europe, I was especially glad to find Raoul Goldberg's confirmation of the insight that there is only one long-term effective way to fight an addictive disposition: the will to become inwardly and outwardly free. He writes: *There is only one power that can save the child's soul and prevent it from sliding into the shadow of dependency and bondage. It is the will to be a free individual. Something within the child must want to be free and to galvanise all those forces of the soul that can help wrest the child from the dark forces of seductive dependency. This power can only come from that free space in the child's being that exists beyond body soul and spirit, that sphere of inner authority and pure activity, in which the choice maker, the integrator, the source and wellspring of our being, the human I, resides.*

As much as every one of us today is in danger of sliding into addictive behaviour, there also lives in each of us just as much a distinctive core to our personality, whose development makes us strong and able to resist such entanglements. That is why we need a concept of health-enhancing schools to move forward. We need schools where the emphasis is on the healthy development of the personality and not just on conveying knowledge or conforming our young people to fit the economic and social mould of modern life. Raoul Goldberg's new book is devoted to this goal, for which he deserves warm thanks on behalf of the younger generations.

Dr Michaela Glöckler
Medical Section at the Goetheanum
Dornach, 22 February 2012

Foreword: A Pandemic in Our Times

The phenomenon of addiction has become one of the most critical socio-cultural problems of our time affecting children as much as adults. Never before has a civilisation been affected by addictive tendencies as is happening today, and never has it affected the children of a civilisation as it is doing in our age. It is regarded by experts in the field of addiction as a serious threat to the health of our children.

In a culture where children are exposed from the earliest age to quick fixes and instant gratification, we are seeing pandemic addictive behaviour and full-on addictions at younger ages than ever before. It is not just dependency on illicit substances that is creating this worldwide pandemic, but also addictions to food and society sanctioned substances (cigarettes, alcohol, caffeine beverages), to electronic gadgetry (computers, cellphones, hand-held devices, game devices), to cybernetworks (internet, social networking, chatrooms), to entertainment media (TV, cinema, audiovisuals) to violence and to excessive and unhealthy sexual practices (pornography, promiscuity, prostitution).

Although each of these addictive agencies have well researched consequences for physical, mental and emotional health which we will investigate in the forthcoming pages, they all in addition have one major deleterious effect in common: namely that the addictive experience itself appears to have a generic human reality of creating subservience and dependency. This will be described in some detail in the first three chapters.

The prevalence of addictive eating disorders such as obesity, anorexia nervosa and bulimia nervosa has increased greatly over the past decade, especially in developed countries. In the USA, at least 15% of children are obese and in South Africa research suggests that 1 in 5 girls has an eating disorder. Twenty percent of American adolescents aged twelve to seventeen are smokers, who are eight times more likely to use illicit drugs and eleven times more likely to drink heavily than non-smoking adolescents. Globally, the highest rate of illicit drug use occurs between eighteen to twenty years (18%), sixteen to seventeen year olds are not far behind (15.6%) and twelve to thirteen year olds make up 4.5%. In South Africa about 10% of high school children use crystal methamphetamine and adolescents constitute about one third of drug rehab patients. It is estimated that in this country between 25% to 43% of sex and violent crimes against children are committed by children themselves – some as young as six years old.

In the short space of a few decades, this phenomenon has begun to change the way many children and youth experience themselves and the world around them; they are becoming progressively alienated from their bodies, from nature, from their fellow human beings, and from their own true potential. At the same time it may be seen as a sign of the times in which these children live, where freedom and self-determination are the evolutionary trends that children and youth are trying to emulate.

This book will explore the inner character of addictive behaviour in children and youth and will offer a tried and tested method to understand each individual child who succumbs to these unhealthy dependencies. From this, a rational approach to helping children with addictive tendencies will be evolved.

We shall see that the phenomena of addiction touch many of us in deep places. Those who in our tasks as parents, teachers and carers of children, have to deal with children and youth caught up with these problems, may be deeply affected by these experiences. We will discover in these pages that the character of addiction is deeply rooted in the human condition and is something that touches everyone to some degree. This means that we all know something about it, giving us a point of departure for our own authentic and original experience. Through our own personal experience we can gain direct access to the range of addictive phenomena that confront us in the world outside. This opens up an empathetic approach to understanding these children, which in turn provides creative opportunities to help children in the most profound ways.

While this book is primarily one about addiction in childhood and adolescence, the core nature of addiction is the same for adults. I deliberated for some time as to whether this book should be focused on childhood addictions, because my approach to this global problem and much of the content of this book, applies as much to adults as to children and adolescents. Furthermore, in my work as a medical practitioner and psychotherapist I see many cases of adult addictions and the need to find ways of helping adult addictions is certainly as urgent as that for children. However, in the end I decided to direct my focus in this book to children and youth because I believe the disposition and the root causes for most addictions in adulthood lie in childhood. Indeed I would go so far as to say that most psycho-emotional problems in adult life have their origins in the childhood years before puberty.

It was the realisation, many years ago, that the primary foundations for health, both on the physical and psychological level, are laid down in the first ten to twelve years, that inspired me to do whatever I could to promote, protect and nurture the health of children in the widest possible way. I dedicated a good part of my professional medical work to treating children and advising parents of their optimal care. I further took up the daunting task of writing about children. I found I could only do this in an authentic way by exploring within myself the journey of my own childhood and adolescent experience. This took place mainly during my training in Psychophonetics Counselling. Psychophonetics is a method of personal transformation and self-development, life coaching, consultancy and psychotherapy based on Rudolf Steiner's anthroposophy and psychosophy, and developed by its founder Yehuda Tagar. It acknowledges the living body, soul and individual spirit as elements of an integral human constitution with a potential connection to vast resources of vitality, creativity, intelligence, compassion, intimacy, expanded awareness and spirituality.[1]

During this training, I discovered that the whole of my childhood and adolescence was present in my unconscious inner life, layered like annual rings in a tree and that it was possible to consciously access this hidden life story. From these personal experiences and from my work as a psychophonetic practitioner, I am convinced that these past experiences lie hidden within us all because we all have been there before, and that with the right interest and proper training we can bring at least some of these experiences to conscious memory. It is not only the content of the past that we can vividly recall, sometimes in great detail, but also the inner personal feelings of what it is to be a three-year-old, a ten-year-old or a fifteen-year-old child.

My first book *Awakening to Child Health I: Holistic Child and Adolescent Development*, describes the healthy development of the child and adolescent from this point of view.[2] It seeks to enable the reader to discover ways of deeply understanding and caring for children, both the children entrusted to one's care as well as one's own inner child. The second volume – *Awakening to Child Health II: Contemporary Health Disturbances in Childhood and Adolescence* – takes up the most prevalent health issues affecting children and youth in our time and indicates an approach to inwardly experiencing, understanding and caring for these conditions. Addiction is one of these issues that, due to its pandemic nature, deserves a whole book on its own.

It needs to be acknowledged that the contents of this book are taken from articles that I wrote for the *South African Journal of Natural Medicine* in 2007–8.[3] The interest that they generated convinced me that they needed to be reproduced in book form.

Each chapter begins with a reflective paragraph that tries to capture the intention that underlines the chapter.

Chapter 1 will explore the common human experience of needs and their gratification that lies at the basis of all addictions. Chapters 2 and 3 will describe an approach to deep understanding and caring of children and adolescents who have allowed themselves to be snared into unhealthy dependency.

Chapters 4 to 11 will address specific addictions with case histories taken from my clinical practice.

Chapter 12 will look at the serious challenge and struggle that children and adolescents with addictive tendencies have to endure.

People today have access to more information about every possible subject under the sun and beyond than they can possibly absorb. Almost all of this information is taken from others who have either experienced it themselves or have derived it from some other source. It is largely this borrowed information that we take on as our own store of knowledge, forgetting that we may have our own rich treasure of personal experience that is more real than any knowledge gained from the experience of others.

It is one of the primary intentions of this book to awaken to an experience of addiction out of the personal experiences that live in each and every one of us. Such authentic experience shall be the true harbinger that enables us to listen with an awakened heart to children with addictions, to understand them and to find the keen interest to help these children in the most effective way possible.

Chapter 1. Awakening to Addictions

I have seen the scourge of addiction and the devastating effects it can have on our children and youth. I have also seen the power of transformation that comes in overcoming this challenge. I am awakening to the nature of addiction. It plays itself out in the human psyche. I wish to explore the common human experience of needs, their gratification and the dependency spectrum in our everyday life.

—

Timothy's story woke me up to the terrible affliction that an addiction can have on the innocent soul of a growing child. It helped me to understand the power of needs that are unfulfilled and the desperate struggle a child may have to endure in order to satisfy these needs.

Timothy was a highly intelligent and sensitive ten-year-old boy, who lost his father tragically in a diving accident. His father, the rock of the family and his major role model, who taught him to surf, advised him on his exercise plan and who was always present when he needed help or advice, was suddenly no longer there for him. Initially, Timothy expressed little emotion but soon began to show signs of anxiety and insecurity. He became quite obsessive about his schoolwork, spending hours every day on getting his homework and projects done perfectly. Once this was finished he would commence his fitness plan, running five kilometres, followed by exercising and push- ups that he would do periodically throughout the day. At supper time he would eat fastidiously, choosing only certain foods and small portions because this way he felt much more comfortable in his body. Before he could go to sleep, he would check the home security and alarm system many times. It was very difficult for him to relax and have fun; he became more and more serious, asocial and depressed.

Over several months I watched this boy becoming totally overwhelmed by his deep inner needs that compelled him to seek short-lived gratification in a range of obsessive and compulsive activities. His whole waking life seemed to revolve around this desperate need to seek relief from intense internal discomfort through these varied compulsive activities.

It was heartbreaking to witness his anguish at being completely controlled by his needs which could only momentarily be satisfied and which required continuous and exhausting mental and physical activity to bring relief. For he himself had come to realise that he was in the grip of something so powerful that it rendered him utterly helpless. With tears streaming down his pain-contorted face, his desperate cry still echoes in my heart: 'I am so exhausted doing this every day but I cannot stop doing it!'

Needs and gratification

The human being, by virtue of his very needy nature, is a *dependent* being. He is dependent on certain basic requirements such as food nutrients, water, air and the right degree of warmth in order that his body continues functioning in a healthy manner. His healthy emotional life is likewise dependent on the fulfilment of a range of psychological needs such as the need to be loved, cared for, touched, acknowledged, to feel worthy, and so on. And on the mental-spiritual level, he needs to express himself as a unique individual, to be creative, discover who he is, and find his life task or to serve others.

Abraham Maslow, a leader in humanistic psychology, described a hierarchical organisation of needs present in everyone. In the course of child development as the more primitive *bodily needs* such as hunger and thirst are satisfied, the more advanced *psychological needs* become the prime motivators. Later in life as these needs are addressed, higher *mental* or *spiritual needs* become relevant.[1,2]

Even a superficial study of human nature will show that needs and their gratification are an intrinsic part of the human condition, expressing themselves in these different arenas of human activity. It seems they are built into the creative design of all living organisms as an innate existential intelligence, linked directly with the will to survive. Needs and their gratification are the means by which the human being maintains, advances and gratifies his existence.

Reflecting on one's own needs, one discovers there are three distinct spheres where needs are constantly striving for their gratification.

Bodily needs

On the physical level, we can observe how our body breathes in air. The respiratory system functions as if it knows it needs oxygen to survive and its function is designed to provide optimal levels under all conditions; exercise increases the need for oxygen and so breathing speeds up; sleep diminishes the need for oxygen and the breathing slows down. The body appears to know when it needs oxygen but it also knows how much it needs at all times; it is able to finely adjust its function according to its needs, thereby maintaining its existence under all conditions.

We thus see that to sustain life and to maintain healthy function, two factors are needed: firstly a *need intelligence* which knows *what* the body needs to survive – oxygen, water, warmth and a host of nutrients – and *how* to get it by instinctively switching on those physiological mechanisms which enable it to acquire what it needs; secondly a highly efficient regulating *gratification intelligence* that knows *when* its needs have been satisfied, switching off or regulating the system to maintain at all times a healthy state of equilibrium.

Instinct and drives

One element of this creative intelligence (needs/gratification) built into the physical organism is *instinct*. A child instinctively knows how to suck on the breast and what to look for to satisfy his hunger without anyone teaching him to do this. He also knows instinctively how to learn to stand upright, to speak and to think. Another element is the *drive* for food, water, oxygen, and warmth; these are powerful biological forces that activate the physiological will to satisfy these biological needs.

Psychological needs

On the psycho-emotional level, we have needs. Consider the things that satisfy you emotionally, that make you feel happy and inwardly comfortable and that you are constantly striving to maintain. Some of these things may appear to satisfy the body – like the need for a cup of coffee, some chocolate or a glass of wine – but they also satisfy the emotional life; we feel gratified emotionally after a satisfying beverage. These create both a pleasurable inner bodily sensation but also a pleasurable feeling experience. One person may need more the physical satisfaction, another more the emotional gratification. Sensation is an experience that involves bodily sense organs; feeling is an experience independent of the body. Our needs may be purely on the feeling level, for instance we have a need to be loved, to be cared for, to be acknowledged. We may yearn for these pleasurable experiences and do all sorts of things in order to gratify this longing.

These experiences of the inner life – sensation, feeling and emotion – are part of what we shall call the *psyche* or the *soul*. It is out of this region that a wide range of needs is constantly striving for their gratification.

In this domain, we observe again a need intelligence which knows what the soul needs for its wellbeing and what it must do to acquire them; we also find a gratification intelligence that in the healthy state will instinctively know when these needs have been gratified. On the other hand, when the neediness for whatever reason cannot be switched off, dependency and addictive behaviour can develop. *It is in the domain of the psyche that the phenomenon of addiction is to be found.*

Desire

The creative intelligence that drives needs in the animal and human psychological organisation is the force commonly called *desire*. It is this force that exerts the most powerful effect on our emotions and feelings, impelling us to seek out the object of our desire. When we meet it, we want it even more intensely and feel satisfied only when we feel we have acquired some of it. We have *desires* for a wide range of objects: for specific foods and drinks, for a cigarette, the newspaper, for sex or for a host of emotional objects. Recall something that you desire intensely and notice where it takes you. The thought of a chocolate may call up sensations or feelings that are only appeased by acquiring it, even if it means going out and buying one in the middle of the night. It is an extraordinary power that takes control of us and forces us to follow the desire. What is this force that can take over our will in such a powerful way, directing our actions to follow its command? It may require an enormous counterforce to oppose this power and a continuous self-regulating activity to keep the force of desire in check. Is it so different in its intensity from the bodily impulse that drives one to drink water to quench one's thirst? In the case of desire, the sphere of action is the human psyche where the focus is not on the preservation of life, but on the degree of comfort and pleasure that can be achieved. Desire is a power of the will that seeks to gratify the needs of the soul. One can readily see how closely connected desire is with the problem of addiction.

Mental-spiritual needs

Thinking and self-reflection create needs that go beyond the volitional, sentient and emotive needs of the psyche. The moment one recognises oneself as a self-contained individual with unique capacities, one discovers one has needs to know something, to become something, to achieve something, to create something. These needs do not arise out of the domain of the body or the psyche, nor does their gratification bring physical or emotional comfort. They belong to another sphere of human activity, which is connected to higher realities, to the sphere of the good and the true. There is a part of every human being that strives for the good and the true. It is this part that we shall call the *higher Self* or *I* that longs, for instance, to become a doctor, a writer or a good father and wishes to be of help to sick people, to share life experiences through writing or to care well for his children. What are these higher aims and objectives that you are seeking to fulfil in your lifetime? For each of us these are entirely individual, being bound up with the core of who we are, with our unique *I*-ness that makes us so utterly different from every other person.

Once again we find a need intelligence which knows what the higher self aspires to for its wellbeing and what it must do to attain it; there also exists a truth intelligence that knows intuitively when these aspirations have been fulfilled. The highest spiritual ideals are those that will take a long time for their fulfilment.

Motivation-wish-intention-resolution

These higher, more conscious, needs call on mental-spiritual capacities that can fulfil these longings. *Motivation* is a force that directs us after self-reflection to act in a particular way. For instance, once I have consciously experienced a healthy body, I will be motivated to maintain my health. *Wish* is a force that underlies motivation. It knows the solution to a problem before it has taken place; it points to a need that still has to be achieved in the future; it is like a powerful beacon of light or an image of hope that points the way forward to fulfilling one's higher goals. My wish for a healthy body strengthens my motivation to achieve this goal. *Intention* is a wish that takes on a clearer and more tangible form. My intention to eat well and exercise regularly brings the future goal that much closer. *Resolve* is the final act of will that will bring the wish and intention into realisation. Now all that remains is to do it.

The will

Needs and the creative intelligence available to bring about their gratification are all part of an ever-present dynamic activity working largely subconsciously in the human constitution on three main levels:

- on a bodily level it preserves structure, function and life itself;
- on a psychological level it provides comfort, pleasure and emotional wellbeing;
- on a spiritual level it fulfils higher longings and aspirations.

This force underlies the very core of our existence and works like a dynamo, energising and activating all other functions. The only word that accurately expresses this activity is the *will,* since we are exercising our will constantly in these activities, either consciously or unconsciously. It is an activity intrinsically bound up with who we are, driving our existence in a very particular way.

Rudolf Steiner first described the anatomy of the will in a course of lectures given to Waldorf teachers in 1919.[3] He indicated that the will is organised in seven different ways, each of which is connected with a different level of the human constitution. As we have seen above, these are:

- instinct, drive   *bodily level*
- desire   *psychological level*
- motivation, wish, intention, resolution   *spiritual level*

Necessity and freedom

On the bodily level there is an absolute necessity to satisfy our biological needs and a very small margin for individual choice. I may be able to withhold my need for oxygen for, at the most, two minutes, but in the end if I am to live, I must continue to breathe; and this is true for everyone.

On the psychological level there are common needs that are also true for everyone, like the need for a child to be loved or cared for, but the intensity of these needs and the quantity required to feel gratified is a personal affair, dependent on a number of external and internal factors related directly to the individual person. There is also a certain level of choice that will determine psychological needs and their gratification. I may wish for warm loving company, but may decide not to enjoy this pleasure for certain reasons.

On the spiritual level, needs and their fulfilment are uniquely individual, whereby each person will exercise a certain degree of freedom and choice in attaining these goals.

The dependency continuum

From the above it can be seen that human needs are an essential part of human existence, serving as the stimulus for the acquisition of the varied elements that will nourish and care for our wholeness and determine our wellbeing. We are dependent on some of these elements; on others we can exercise our choice and free will. The body is completely dependent on a variety of physical and chemical factors for its existence. In exploring the phenomenon of addiction, we are obviously not concerned with the dependency of the body on such life-sustaining elements like air and water. On the other side, the higher Self has a large measure of independence where it can make choices that at least are free of the body and the psycho-emotional impulses and activities. This would appear to be the domain of self-regulation and self-control, which we shall draw on actively in the management of addiction. *It is in the domain of the psyche that the phenomenon of addiction plays itself out, where a dependency of the soul life may express itself through a compulsive urge, craving or longing to satisfy an inner emotional need.*

Dependency

The Oxford Dictionary defines addiction as the process of *being dependent on something*, of being unable to do without something. It comes from the word *addicere* meaning to assign, or appoint: that is, the *addict* is assigned or compelled to something to which he becomes dependent. Although the term addiction is not considered a scientific term, having become trivialised by common usage and stigmatised by the negative and emotive connotation it conjures up, I have chosen to retain the term to refer to that extreme form of dependence along the dependency life curve.

23

Experiencing addictive tendencies

We all have our likes and dislikes, certain things cause us pleasure and comfort, other things create displeasure and discomfort. We usually strive to attain what gives us pleasure and makes us comfortable and we can become quite attached to such comforts. Recall what gives you special pleasure: reading the newspaper, watching the stock exchange, smoking a cigarette, enjoying your morning coffee, relaxing with a glass of wine, watching a TV series.

We may notice that our need for this pleasure can become more intense when we are upset or irritated by something and we may then go out of our way to re-experience the pleasure; and when we are not able to enjoy it, we may feel quite put out, as if something is missing in our lives. How does it feel when you miss your habitual comfort or pleasure?

Many of our habits arise out of specific needs and inclinations and when these habits alter we may notice some discomfort. Our needs are then no longer met and our need intelligence tells us something is wrong. Until we realise where the need is coming from and search for a more healthy way of dealing with it, we shall have to admit that we are dependent on this habitual activity to gratify our specific need. But why search for something else to satisfy your need when a cigarette, or exercising or even the desire to help someone, does the job? It is common human behaviour to stubbornly hold on to that which gives us comfort, satisfaction and fulfilment.

On the basis of specific biological and psychological needs, we construct unconsciously, during the first phase of our life, learned ways of thinking, feeling and behaving to which we become habituated: perfectionist behaviour makes one feel more in control; reactive behaviour patterns such as withdrawal in the face of criticism are mechanisms of self-defence. To some degree we become dependent on these personality traits, behaviour patterns or activities.

There are certain substances and activities that the body or mind gets used to, resulting in higher quantities or frequent repetition being needed to produce the same effect. This is called *tolerance*. If the substance or activity is suddenly stopped, physical or psychological discomfort occurs, a condition known as *withdrawal*. The body or the mind has now become seriously dependent or addicted to the substance or activity. At this point the person can no longer resist the desire to gratify his need and the gratification agency becomes like a dictator, compelling the

24

needy one to engage and satisfy his need. Addiction develops when the gratification becomes too powerful to resist and the person loses the self-determination to decide what is good for him. The self then becomes the slave to the tyrannical addiction.

I believe most of us have experienced some degree of compulsive or addictive behaviour whereby our desire took on a life of its own and where, for a period of time, we were no longer directed by our more rational self.

Our struggle between gratification and self-control

When we attentively observe human behaviour, our own or others, we will recognise that one part of our nature is hell bent on gratifying our needs and desires, while another part has the ability to control these needs according to our rational thinking. Some of the time our emotional needs get the upper hand; other times our rational mind keeps us on track. We play out a life long struggle between wanting to gratify our lower soul nature and controlling this with our higher human resources, a struggle that takes place in the realms we may call the psyche and the higher Self. When the needs of the soul are too strong, the self-regulating balancing force of the Self may not be able to contain its power. Steiner called this struggle the *main game* of human evolution and it is within this *life spectrum of dependency* that addictive behaviour needs to be understood.[4]

In the next chapter we will explore more deeply the nature of addiction and in particular, the way it affects children and youth.

Chapter 2. Understanding Addiction in Children and Young Adults

Every encounter I have with childhood addiction enters my experience and becomes a part of my inner life. This inner experience becomes my starting point to understand this phenomenon. From here I wish to find a way to deepen my understanding of addictions in childhood and adolescence so that I may know about it from inside. I will then be able to meet and address this challenging phenomenon of the modern age that affects each and every one of us.

—

There is no better way of understanding dependency and addiction than by starting with our own personal experience.

Encounter with addictive tendencies in children

In many socially and economically unstable communities, such as in the city of Cape Town, it is quite a common experience to encounter street children from six to twelve years of age begging at traffic lights. These are commonly children addicted to alcohol, glue sniffing, methamphetamine, crack or heroin, trying to survive with handouts or by selling their bodies. Equally, many of us are in contact with children who are completely dependent on their mobile phones or spend hours on their computers playing games, surfing the internet or locked away in chat rooms. We see more and more obese children who are addicted to overeating, to sugary foods or cola drinks.

Notice what happens inside of you when you hear about such children or encounter adolescents who appear to be dependent on some addictive agency. You may observe a feeling of sadness, guilt, anxiety or some other discomfort, and an accompanying sensation in your body. Or thoughts and mental pictures may arise about the child, or about some previous experiences related to children or addictions; thoughts and memories about your own personal life may arise, someone you know personally who is addicted to something. Or your own compulsive tendencies may surface. You may be moved to want to do something or to directly react to the child who has been playing computer games for the past three hours. We will all have our own immediate experience of addiction in the moment we encounter the outer world of addiction; the inner world is immediately activated and we take into our personal world this outer impression. The world of addiction that we experienced outside now lives inside and is awakened, even for a moment.

Taking hold of this inner experience of addiction, one can apply a hands-on approach that involves our direct experience with the problem. Out of my working with children and parents over several decades and my training in Psychophonetics, I have evolved a method of awakening to a deeper experience of oneself which can be applied to the encounter with children and their difficulties (see Appendix 2).[1]

An experiential approach to understanding and caring for children

We can focus on any problem that a child might have in one of two ways: we either focus on the outer problem of the child, or we can focus on ourselves and what is evoked in us by confronting the outer issue. Most of the time these two loci of experiences are mixed together, going from one to the other and causing much confusion and distress to all concerned.

A mother may indeed think she is dealing with her child Thomas, who spends hours on the computer, when she screams in frustration at him to stop using it, but in reality she is acting out her own hurt and anger without realising it.

It is not too difficult to learn the skill of focusing first on one's own inner experience and responses, acknowledging who or what is happening there, and dealing with one's own issues. For instance, when Thomas' mother has learnt to self-reflect and examines her own inner experience of reacting to Thomas, she discovers someone inside herself who feels unacknowledged and unheard; her child's disobedience simply adds more to her longstanding hurt, and triggers her frustration and anger. Or she may be in touch with her sense of fear and powerlessness to change his behaviour, linking her to her own history of fear and powerlessness. When she deals lovingly with her inner hurt and soothes the pain, she is only then able to focus properly on her child without her own stuff getting in the way. She may realise through her own previous reflection that Thomas may also feel hurt, unacknowledged and unheard and for this reason spends hours on his chat sites, gratifying his need to be acknowledged and heard. This insight may give her the empathy and the interest to want to relate to the child in a completely different way. She can now turn her focus on her child and observe him as keenly as possible.

Most of us are unskilled in careful observation and unaccustomed in utilising even a small part of our perceptive potential. However, with focus and application, we can all learn to make fuller use of our sensory faculties, thereby enhancing the flow of information coming to us from the outside world. The approach I have developed, called *Awakening to Deep Experience*, is simply to learn to observe the multi-faceted aspects of the object, in this case Thomas, and apply our thinking, feeling, sensing and expressive abilities to discovering consciously as much as possible about the object under scrutiny.

Thomas' mother can turn her attention to looking at multiple ways in which Thomas expresses himself. The appearance of his body, skin, eyes, the warmth of his hands, and his smell, tell a story about his physical nature (physical profile). His particular gestures and the way he moves his body reveal more about his inner character (kinesthetic profile). The manner of his speech, his tonal qualities and modulations, allows his mother to sense his heartfelt feelings and to sense deeply his inner narrative (auditory-tonal profile). The way he forms his thoughts and his unique individuality inform her further about his inner nature (thought-ego profile).

Most people, with a little training, can learn to observe clearly what they perceive and to arrive at a cognitive-sensory picture that provides a great deal of insight into the child's nature. If one wishes to go deeper, one may train oneself further and connect more deeply with the child by employing the skill that young children use unconsciously, and that actors and mimers use consciously – that of *imitation*. Thomas' mother can learn to slip into his skin and, for a short while, play the part of Thomas, becoming Thomas as well as she can, knowing much about him from her previous observations. Once she has experienced Thomas in this way, she can withdraw back into her own self and observe the way she had acted out this role. She had tried to become Thomas, through imitation, by gesturing, moving or speaking like him and now, outside, she observes imaginatively how this after-image looks to her. It is as if she had taken a video clip of herself acting out Thomas, and was now looking at it.

This dramatic action, combined with the observational picture-profile, will enable Thomas' mother to gain new insight and perspective into Thomas as a person and to consider rationally and intuitively how best she can help him. In order to do this she will need to find the best part of herself to manage the problem more effectively. She therefore evokes the most caring attentive mother who is able to listen and respond to her child in ways that make him feel completely heard and understood.

Such an approach can lead to deep understanding and effective caring for both adult carer and child, and can improve relationships in remarkable ways. I refer readers to my book *Awakening to Child Health I*, as well as to Appendix 2 of this book, which utilises this approach in understanding and caring for children both in health and ill health.[2]

This methodology was developed out of Psychophonetics, a method of self-awareness and transformation applied to counselling, coaching, consultancy, parenting and medical practice.[3]

Some people will intuitively be able to employ some aspects of this approach in their interactions with children, whereas other elements will require in-depth training and coaching; entering deeply into the child's inner life will always demand the highest ethical standards.

Approach to children with addictive tendencies

I have found the method described above to be an effective approach to the problem of addictions in childhood and adolescence.

Let us say I encounter a teenager like Sarah who confesses to me that she has been cutting herself for the past three years and has told no one about it. She is not yet willing to see a counsellor and she has only just come to the point of confiding in someone about her compulsive behaviour. How can we best understand and help her?

First and foremost is our willingness to help Sarah; then if we are to really comprehend her predicament, we will need to put aside our own preconceptions, prejudices and emotional blocks by examining our inner response and inner experience to the problem, as indicated above.

Once the inner slate has been cleared, we shall need to find within ourselves a deep interest and respect for Sarah and her difficulties. We shall need to evoke the skills for mindfulness and empathy.

Next we deepen our observational skills by focusing our undivided attention on every sensory impression that Sarah offers us, to create a cognitive-sensory picture in the way described above.

We can then enter this picture empathetically by employing the skill of conscious imitation. We slip into Sarah's skin for a brief period by imitating how we imagine she must feel; we sense and feel our experience of her, then physically gesture our interpretation of what she is experiencing; we hold this gesture for a few moments and then move out of this position by stepping away. We then observe our after-image as well as we can. This psychophonetic technique, called *enter-exit-behold*, allows for a deep insight into Sarah's addictive disposition.[4]

Holistic child and adolescent development

A further element needed in our quest to understand addictions in childhood and adolescence, is a basic working knowledge of the healthy development of a child in her development to adulthood. A short outline of this journey will be described below, but for more detail, I refer readers to my aforementioned book that goes into this subject in much greater depth.

To grasp this journey in its fullness, we will need to have a clear picture of what constitutes a child's whole being. Starting with our own conscious experience, we may explore within ourselves what constitutes the adult human being, knowing that we grew through all the stages of childhood and adolescence to become the adult that we are.

In Chapter 1 we explored the nature of needs and gratification and found that these were related to three different realms of our existence. We have physical needs for food, drink, oxygen and warmth to sustain our *body,* and our physical organisation is designed to procure the life giving elements until the need for them has been satisfied. We also have psychological needs such as the need to be loved, cared for, stimulated and respected to sustain our *psyche,* and our psychological organisation will do everything in its power to gratify these needs. We also saw that we have mental and spiritual needs related to higher aspirations and goals, which sustain our spirit, such as the wish to do good in the world and to become an honest and trustworthy human being; our mental and spiritual life possesses the capacities to makes these dreams and wishes come true.

We may discover that fundamentally there are three distinct aspects that make up every human being:

- There is a part that belongs to the given world of nature, that contains all the physical and chemical components of the outer world, and that can be perceived by the physical senses as an outer object. We call this the *body,* which is made up of all kinds of solid, liquid, gaseous and warm parts.
- Then there is an organised inner world of experience that embraces our psychological functions of cognitive activities, feeling responses, perceptions and sensations and willed actions. We can name this the *psyche* or *soul* . This follows laws that are quite different to the laws that govern matter.
- Finally, there is a part of our being that goes beyond our personal character with its likes and dislikes and belongs to a more universal reality that has to do with what is true and good. We can call this the *spirit,* which is subject to laws that are again quite different to those of the body and the psyche.

Working through all three domains of human existence, it is the unique individuating power of who we are, the *Self* or *I,* which stands at the core of every human being, which integrates and holds our whole being together and which carries our higher intentions and destiny like a guiding star throughout our life.

We can observe that, during life, these three aspects are interconnected in a continuum that determines every aspect of our being. For instance when the needs of the body are paramount, say when we feel hungry, our psycho-spiritual functions may take a back seat until the hunger is satisfied. Our desire for a particular food may drive our body a long way to acquire it. Yet the motivation and resolve to resist this food will stop both body and psyche from exerting its influence over our spiritual nature.

We further discover that the soul lies between the body and spirit, given that part of its nature is closely connected with the body, while another part is connected with the spirit. Sensation is a function of the soul that is rooted in the body, and requires physical sense organs to operate, while thinking is an aspect of the soul life that serves the spirit. Through thinking we can choose not to gratify our desires. The soul mediates between the body that is oriented towards the physical earthly domain, and the spirit that comes from and is directed towards spiritual dimensions.

The child's emerging soul likewise exists and develops between the body and spirit.

We may depict the body-soul-spirit continuum in the following way:

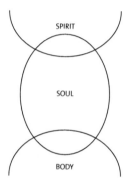

Figure 1. Body-soul-spirit continuum in the human being.

For the first period of life, the child is dependent to a large degree on her environment for the gratification of her needs. In the first nine months, the growing embryo is developing inside the embryonic sheaths of its mother's body; it is completely dependent on this body for all its physical and biological needs. Indeed the very first physical germinal cells, the sex cells that united at conception to form the original embryonic germ cell, are derived from the parents. The child's body needs to attain a certain level of physical maturity before it can be born as an independent physical body that no longer requires the mother's sheaths for its every bio-physical need. Yet this body at birth is primarily inherited from and therefore dependent on her parents and her fore-fathers and -mothers.

During the next seven years, every cell of the body, which the child inherited, will be replaced by cells and tissues that she herself produces. In other words, the child is actively transforming and re-modelling this inherited body into one that she can call her own and that will be suitable for her life journey. During this time, when the child's biological functions are dynamically at work in creating her own unique biological organisation, she is still dependent on her parents, especially the carer that nourishes and cares for her basic needs: food, water, warmth, care and protection. Needs that she cannot herself provide, she requires her carers to provide for her. It is as if her own biological functions are pre-occupied with other work, and require to be protected by the bio-functional sheaths of her carers, just as her physical body was previously protected by the embryonic sheaths of her mother. We can recognise when this process comes to an end, usually in the seventh year, when the hardest tissues – the teeth – are ejected because they are too hard to be transformed internally. At this time we can observe a decisive change in the child: she becomes more self-sufficient, helping herself to food, dressing with the right clothes and preparing herself for school. She gradually begins to shake off the biological sheath of her carers, as if she was being born a second time. This takes the best part of seven years to come to fruition and it is imperative for the healthy development of the child's biological functions that during this time the very best support for these functions can be given.

At the same time as the physical body is growing and transforming, the psychological functions are awakening and developing. It is in the nature of the human being that there is a close correspondence between physiological functions and psychological activities. The first activities to show themselves in the newborn child are primitive *will* functions in the sense described above: the child grows from her instincts and drives that impel her forward and enable all her developmental milestones to unfold in a highly predictable manner. The will to explore the world activates and drives the next soul activities – her sensory faculties which then have no bounds. It is as if the whole child becomes a sense organ and she instinctively learns the art of imitation through sensing and feeling herself into everything that confronts her in the outer world. It is her neuro-sensory apparatus that must develop quickly and preferentially to support these functions. During this period these soul functions are bound up with the body and express themselves through physiological functions. Thus the feelings of anxiety in a child may manifest as tummy aches or skin rashes.

Between seven and fourteen years, her capacity to have feelings independent of the bodily needs unfolds. Now it is no longer hunger or thirst that determines her wellbeing; instead, she now feels intensely when her best friend wants to play with another girl. Her bodily functions are no longer affected by emotions as they were before. It is also no coincidence that during this period the rhythmically functioning organs like the heart, lungs and all other bio-rhythmic activities are growing and maturing. For these rhythms, embracing as they do the polarities of contraction and expansion, as in the beat of the heart or the breathing in and out of the lung, provide the physiological basis for the psychological function of feeling. The feeling-life likewise contains extremes like joy and sorrow, love and hate and all their gradations, as well as an activity that can hold these extremes through the power of balance and harmony. It is this journey into the life of feelings that the child during these years must travel, to explore all the varied nuances of feelings and to learn how to activate the harmonising power that can balance them out.

While this is happening, her tender soul life is awakening as it were from a slumbering gestation deep within the body, and needs the right care and protection from those individuals close to her. Initially she relies mainly on her immediate care givers, but later her school teachers may play a greater role. She gradually finds her own community of friends and comrades who, more and more, take over from her close care givers. This is why the group psyche – the gang, fashions and fads, the best friends, and so on – will feature prominently in the child's life, representing as it does the soul life of the primary school child until she comes of age. It is as if her emerging soul life needs to be held from the outside in a kind of communal soul sheath until it is strong and robust enough to venture out independently into the outer world. This happens around the time of *puberty*, in which we can recognise, by the wide range of prominent physical and psychological changes, that a new child has been born. A third birth has taken place, that of her independent and self-contained soul life.

It will be readily understood that with the awakening of the soul, the child enters another critical phase of her development. She is now less vulnerable to her biological needs which she can, to a certain degree, take care of, but she is still highly vulnerable to her psychological needs because she is not yet mature enough to provide for them. This is to be expected since she is working on the construction of a healthy soul organisation in the same way that the embryo was building a physical body within the warmth and protection of her mother's body. Her unprotected soul life, wherein her desires, sensitivity, sensuality, sexuality, emotionality and feelings reside, is therefore especially vulnerable to the psycho-emotional impressions she receives from her environment. The kind of psycho-social environment in which the child grows up, in the thirteen or fourteen years up to puberty, will play a critical role in the healthy development of the psyche.

If the psychological needs of a child are not met during this period, the child will be at risk of seeking her gratification in unhealthy ways. *One can therefore predict that when the psycho-social environment of a child is sub-optimal, that this will be the time when the seeds for addictive behaviour are laid down.*

With the threshold reached at puberty, the child takes a mighty step forward in her development. Just as the change of teeth expresses the closure of one developmental period and the liberation of a growth process in another area, so puberty testifies to the conclusion of a second life epoch and the awakening of new developmental activities that determine the future direction of the child's life.

Growth is now directed preferentially to the metabolic, uro-genital and musculo-skeletal systems; the sexual organs develop, accompanied by growth in the larynx in boys, chest and limbs. At the same time her awakened soul life opens itself to new experiences – to her sexuality, to heightened emotionality and to a new capacity of rational thinking. She becomes conscious of her new emerging strengths: on the one hand the physical power of her developing body, on the other new powers of the soul that allow her to open herself more safely to the outside world. She discovers her growing independence and with it a greater measure of control over her environment.

In the period between puberty and adulthood, when physical growth of the body ceases in the twentieth year, we can witness momentous manifestations of the liberated soul life. Powerful emotions awaken through the force of desire as well as the experiencing of deep feelings like shame, anger, love, hate and despair. They are accentuated by a newly awakened sense of movement and passion brought about by the surge of hormones and the growth of limbs; there is a need to dance, to compete in sports, to do martial arts, to travel. Alongside these strong feelings, the power of fantasy begins to grow as a flow of wish-filled mental pictures that create her ideal future. This may lead to her first real love for another person, to adventures and dangerous exploits, to her choice of career or to following her passion for the highest ideals.

On the other hand, the young adolescent may feel as if she has been thrown out into a hostile world, where she feels alone and exposed. She may withdraw into her inner private world because she feels unheard and misunderstood. If her education does not meet her needs, if her community or social activities do not provide her with the necessary psycho-spiritual support or if no person takes an interest in trying to understand this young individual, she can become too self-absorbed in her own problems, leading to all kinds of unfavourable outcomes. *The most common of these will be addictive tendencies.*

The teenager and adolescent requires to be held quietly and respectfully by the social community that surrounds her, while she is developing her identity as a unique individual. She will be grappling with questions and issues that her awakened thinking throws at her: who am I in myself? Who am I in relation to others? Who am I in relation to the world and my life path? It is as if she is digesting and discovering herself consciously while at the same time facing the world on her own. It is critical to understand that the soul's awakening during these years will bring with it all kinds of difficulties and enormous challenges for the young person. It is therefore imperative that she experiences the support of her social community and individual mentors who provide her with an invisible protective sheath while she is working out her individual life. It is only around the age of twenty, when she receives symbolically the key to her own free life, that she throws off this protective sheath and emerges as a self-contained individual person, mature enough to run and organise her life the way she sees fit.

The nature of addiction

We have set the stage for an understanding of the phenomenon of addiction. We have examined needs and gratification and the problem of dependency as key factors leading to the core of addictions. We have an approach to experiencing and understanding addictions at a deep level. And we have outlined the fundamental features of child and adolescent development during which time it is probably true to say that all, or at least most, addictions have their origin.

With this as a background let us now look at the nature of the addictive phenomenon itself, in particular in the way it affects children and adolescents.

Normal child development follows distinct and predictable stages where development of the body, soul and spirit are inextricably bound up and finely synchronised with one another. The specific needs of each domain will make themselves felt and will seek their natural gratification within the normal developmental process. We have also seen how the different dimensions of the child's being are embedded in the environmental sheaths of parental home, school community and social grouping, which should provide the natural and healthy means of fulfilling these needs.

There are fundamental needs, as described above, which belong to the growing and evolving human being. We never stop growing and we never stop having real needs. Real needs such as the need for love, warmth, safety, being touched, acknowledged, appreciated and respected, long to be satisfied. Children, by their very nature, want and expect their needs to be gratified and suffer acutely when their core needs are not met; a hungry child will tell you in no uncertain terms that she needs to eat, for the body needs food to grow; the biological need intelligence knows that without food the body will perish. In the same way a neglected child will feel the intense discomfort of an absent mother, and will also act out her discomfort in some obvious way. The psyche too knows that it needs the soul nourishment of being nurtured and protected in order for it to grow in a healthy way; it will wither if it does not receive this and many other soul needs.

Unfortunately, too often a child's natural environment does not provide this. Parents are unable or unwilling to give the child what she needs; or the child, for a variety of inner reasons is unable to absorb it; for instance a three-year-old child may feel threatened by the arrival of a new born sibling, become aggressive and defiant and begin to eat her own faeces.

Children do not have the psychological resilience to resist gratifying their needs nor to distinguish healthy from unhealthy gratification; they cannot easily talk themselves out of the need to be loved and acknowledged because it is their right to receive this and somewhere deep within they know this. And so these needs do not go away. The grave danger is that their natural real needs can be claimed and subverted by other enticements that latch on to these needy children. This is why children are so vulnerable to addictive agencies.

Psychodynamics of addiction

But how does the addictive dependency arise in the first place? Can we enter empathically into the soul experience of a child, and discover the inner dynamics that lead to dependency?

Pandora, who is fifteen years of age, is addicted to crack cocaine. His parents both work full time and have been too busy with their own issues to take much interest in his life. Whenever he finds himself under pressure at home or school he finds comfort and refuge in snorting this drug. But his relief is short-lived and is usually followed with guilt, shame and bouts of depression. The only way he can finance the drug is to become a dealer; he becomes caught in a world of blackmail, deceit, subterfuge and fear. He has constant nasal problems, is constantly fighting with his parents and his performance at school is deteriorating.

When we are able to put aside our own issues for a brief while and live into the experience of this boy, what do we discover? *A deeply anxious and needy child who has found a false substitute for the comfort and caring that his absent parents are unable to give him.*

Deeper exploration reveals the following: it is very uncomfortable, even painful, for Pandora to be deprived of his core primary needs. At some point in time, the discomfort or pain becomes too much for him and he gives up on these needs, suppressing them to halt the pain. This creates a primary block to the need. The acute pain may be appeased, but the barrier to the original need causes a kind of congestion or constriction in his psyche leading to psychological discomfort that takes the form of anxiety, craving and negativity of various kinds. Once again Pandora cannot stand this soul irritation. He cannot bear the pain or discomfort of what is missing. He may attempt to deal with it by making use of defence mechanisms such as avoidance and compensations of various kinds. Eventually, he adopts a secondary substitute, in the form of crack cocaine that gives relief to the discomfort.

The needy child will search for any means to gratify his needs and can easily be sucked into whatever gives comfort to the needy soul, a habit, a substance or a particular behaviour pattern. Thus the addiction to some substance or activity is found that now attaches itself to the psychological domain where needs and gratification resides – overshadowing and influencing all levels of the will that have been previously described: instinct, drives, desires, motivation, wish, intention and resolve. And the more the child feeds the habit, the bigger it becomes.

Whereas real needs are always eventually satisfied and are governed by a sense of moderation and proportion, acquired needs can never be satisfied and never satisfy the real needs. They become invasive and controlling like some foreign agents of the soul, using the energy of the real needs to achieve their goal.

All addictions, whether they are food, sanctioned or illicit substances, media, electronic addictions, violence or sexual aberrations, manage to get in and take hold because they are able to soothe or numb the irritation of the basic needs that are not being met. They may be regarded as the result of blocked or suppressed real needs; they are the adoption of a damaging habit in response to a secondary need that is always a substitute for a real need which has been blocked (see box).[3,4,5]

> Unfulfilled primary need → pain → blocking of the need → ensuing congestion and discomfort → the finding and adopting of a substitute gratification → appeases the pain briefly → secondary need → dependency on substitute agency

Addictive partnership

How is it possible that the need for something is so powerful that the addict repeatedly seeks for it, even though it may be so damaging? Why do Pandora or Timothy in Chapter 1, continue to compulsively gratify their needs, even though they know only too well how destructive it is for them and those around them?

When we enter the inner nature of addiction we always encounter two components: a powerful *addictive compelling or tempting force* that imposes a certain action on another *helpless, submissive, suffering recipient,* whose discomfort is invariably appeased by receiving this offering. There is a needy person in Pandora who desperately seeks to appease his discomfort no matter at what cost; but there is also a person who compels him or tempts him into repeatedly giving in to the gratification of his needs.

A silent contract is playing itself out in this partnership where the passive receiver is so needy for what the active partner has to give, that she agrees to give up everything to receive it; however the need, the craving can never be satisfied. It is never enough. All she gets is a short period of pleasure or respite from discomfort where her stress and tensions are removed. The addict learns to rely on the addiction for comfort from pain, for nurturing or relief from stress. But at what a price!

All addicts are aware of this deep down; they know that their self-worth and integrity are compromised; their health and energy suffers; their time, finances and human relationships are sacrificed, and their freedom is taken away. They are very aware that their will to stop the habit is very weak. The more they use it, the more the addiction grows; they have lost control over their ability to say no and to make choices. Their behaviour is part of a cycle of thinking, feeling and acting which they cannot control. The cycle brings despair, degradation, shame and danger.

The environment of addiction

Why has addictive behaviour in children become so widespread today?

The environment modern children find themselves in has changed dramatically, reflecting the evolving nature of humanity. The present times are characterised by a search for self-identity and self-determination. Even in their need to conform, modern adolescents feel themselves as unique individuals searching for their rightful place in the world. The child is losing, at an ever earlier age, the natural environmental support of parents, community, religion and traditions. She seeks elsewhere for her support and for the gratification of her needs; she finds comfort and satisfaction in her *social peer group, in the virtual reality of the world media, and in the power and seduction of the electronic age.*

Her peer group provides her with a sense of belonging where she can safely explore her self-identity and determine her particular way of gratifying her personal needs. It is here that she will frequently find the moral justification for her protest against the modern world, her healthy need to liberate herself from her parents and her longing for the intoxication of threshold experiences such as drugs, sex, violence and extreme sports that cut through one-sided attachments to the material world.

The world media create a ready-made sensational virtual reality of life through which she tries, in her fantasy, to satisfy her deepest inner needs.

And the electronic age provides the child with a megalomanic sense of her own power; she can create, control, gratify her desires instantly through the press of a button. She has the feeling of invincibility and being able to determine her own destiny. And she can do all this in the privacy of her home, without having to confront the outer world

It is into this seductive environment that lonely and insecure children and youth, who have underlying emotional issues such as self-doubt, poor self-esteem and anxiety, compounded by environmental stresses such as poverty, abuse, parental separation, unemployment, family death or illness in the family, will find refuge.

A large proportion of children will explore the exhilarating freedom of these three fields of experience (peer group, media and electronics) as the natural adventurism of youth. The unhealthy nature of many of these experiences are usually not seriously damaging to health. Some children, however, whose inner needs are so great and who find constant gratification in substitutive substances or behaviour patterns are hooked into a potentially highly damaging way of life which threatens every aspect of their lives.

Some of these children and young adults will abuse substances or agencies in ways that may be extremely harmful to their lives, yet they do not become addicts. Only a small percentage become addicted to the point where there is a compulsive dependency or craving for something which cannot be resisted, where higher quantities or frequent repetition become necessary to produce the same effect and where withdrawal symptoms occur when the substance or agency is suddenly stopped. These are the young people who become alienated from the world, from their fellow human beings and from the greater part of themselves.

The addictive brain

We may well ask what role the brain plays in the causation of addiction.

If the cause is a defect in brain chemistry or brain function, then theoretically the addiction could be overcome if normal brain chemistry could be restored, just as a diabetic patient can live a normal life when treated with insulin. This would fit with the mainstream 'Disease Model of Illness' that regards all illness as a specific physical or chemical defect in some organ or biological system and that leads to a set of signs and symptoms in the patient.[6] Biomedical addiction specialists have, for decades, regarded addiction as a disease like any other physical illness, and in recent years high-tech neuro-imaging and neuropharmacology has been able to identify what neuroscience believes is the physical defect of addiction and where in the brain it occurs.[7,8] It appears to occur in a part of the brain that handles core survival experience, known as the *limbic brain* or more exactly the part called the *ventral tegmentum* and *amygdala*. This is a section of the brain that experiences desire, pleasure and wellbeing and which has a great deal to do with our fundamental survival instincts. In addiction the defect is believed to be a dysfunction in the limbic-dopamine system leading to deregulation of the experience of desire and the sense of pleasure. The symptoms that seem to be associated with this dysfunctional reward system are loss of control, craving and persistent drug use despite negative consequences. The drug becomes the vehicle for survival and when it is unavailable the addict craves it as if he were craving life itself.

Dopamine is commonly associated with those parts of the brain called the *hedonic* or *reward system* which seem to regulate and control behaviour. It seems to do this by inducing desire, pleasurable effects and feelings of anticipation that reinforce behaviour to proactively perform certain activities. Almost all addictive drugs act upon the brain's reward system to increase dopamine release. Food, sex, and other naturally rewarding experiences also release dopamine.

Dopamine is not, however, simply the pleasure-inducing chemical in the brain; it is also released when negative stimuli such as pain or aggression are encountered or when a reward is greater than anticipated. For this reason, some researchers think it may be related to desire rather than pleasure. This may explain why drugs like antipsychotics, that inhibit dopamine activity, reduce people's desire for pleasure, but don't make that pleasure less intense.[9]

Since *craving* is the fundamental experience common to all addiction, it would seem plausible that dopamine has something to do with craving, a psychosomatic experience that is directly connected with desire. In Chapter 1 we described desire as a will-based experience, which explains why craving is such a powerful, wilful and body-based experience.

As the addict continues to overstimulate this reward circuit, the brain has to adapt by producing less of the hormones. This decrease compels those addicted to the dopaminergic-effect of the drug, to increase the drug consumption in order to re-create the earlier or initial experiences and to bring their 'feel-good' hormone level back to normal, leading to tolerance of the drug. Removal of the drug drops the neuro-hormones to sub-survival level with concomitant withdrawal symptoms. Modern antipsychotics are designed to block dopamine function. Unfortunately, this blocking can also cause relapses into depression, and increases in addictive behaviours.

This disease model theory places the cause of addiction solely and firmly in the arena of the body. Inconveniently, however, it confronts experience that does not seem to be of a bodily nature, phenomena which are characterised as mental, emotional and spiritual in nature.

Pandora had every intention of trying to stop his cocaine addiction. He resolved many times to stop and vowed over and again that this would be the last time. Every time he succumbed he was overcome with guilt and shame. When he found compassion for himself and learned how to start valuing and caring for himself, a new life opened for him. He slowly but surely found his way back to normal physical and mental health.

On the basis of common human experience we have described the three aspects that constitute the human being: a sense perceptible *body* that contains all the physical and chemical components of the outer world, a *soul* or *psyche* that embraces our inner world of experience, and a *spirit* that belongs to a universal reality that transcends body and soul. We may also experience our *I* or *higher Self* as the eternal core of our being that holds everything together in an integrated whole.

This separation between the sense-perceptible bodily realm and the supersensible psycho-spiritual realm has been a very inconvenient reality for biomedical science ever since René Descartes enunciated his dualistic conception of mind and body in the seventeenth century. This theory, which holds that the mental realm is a completely different and quite separate reality from the bodily realm, obviously contradicts our daily reality where we see mind and body constantly meeting and interacting with one another. It has had significant consequences in the medical field. For instance, mental illnesses were not accorded the same status as physical illnesses and medical science has not known quite how to explain experiences such as *consciousness, compassion, love* or *enthusiasm*. That is until neuro-physiology or neuro-chemistry discovered areas in the brain where some correlation with these experiences was shown to exist. When

43

an experience of exultation or joy could be consistently highlighted by neuro-imaging in a specific area of the brain, it was persuasive to believe that here was the source of exultation and joy in the human being.

One way of solving this mind/body problem was simply to say that consciousness was a feature of the physical organisation of the brain, so that our mental characterisations are simply physical descriptions on another level.[10] Thus the *experience* of 'wetness' is an expression of the 'physical interaction between water molecules', on another level. 'Thus, the mental and the physical are really the same thing'.[11] Such a viewpoint removes any confusion between mental and physical, between mental disorder and physical disorder, and addiction can now simply be regarded as a defect in the brain's ability to perceive pleasure, forcing the addict to form a pathological attachment to the drug.

There is only one problem with this theory: it does not accord with our human experience; apart from this it makes a mockery of the human being as a free spirit. Biomedical science would have us believe that the highest human experiences – what we name as *I, Soul* and *Spirit* and what we create for the higher good – is like everything else in our systems, a kind of material product of the body, like a neuro-chemical secretion or a creation of the human genome. Such a viewpoint, in my opinion, subjugates and demeans the highest human reality to a factor determined by the material world. In this scenario there would be no possibility of human freedom. The greatest human discoveries, creativity and expressions of moral rightness such as love, loyalty and goodness would all have to be regarded as material products of the body. The human being would have no free choice and there would be no choice of freedom. Yet our experience tells us that we do have choices. We can decide to oppose needs and desires of the body and soul, such as addictive tendencies, and act in a way that we believe is good and true. We discover, in so doing, that we have the potential for freedom.

The body-soul-spirit continuum

Our human experience tells us that there is a constant interplay between the activities of the body, soul and spirit. We can all remember experiences that link emotions and bodily functions. What happens within your body when you are angry, frustrated, worried, enthusiastic or excited? How do you feel emotionally when your body aches from flu? What happens when you override a craving for chocolate, knowing that you have had enough?

This pneumo-psychosomatic continuum can be viewed as the human reality upon which health, illness and healing rests.[1] The idea that the soul and spirit are independent entities, not part of the body, is difficult for Western bioscience to conceive because this cannot be proven according to the modern scientific method. (Before the discovery of magnetism, it was also difficult to imagine that invisible force fields could inhabit physical bodies.)

Once one conceives the psyche and spirit as independent, highly organised force fields that interact with the physical/functional body, one will not have to postulate monistic materialistic theories that regard the human being as a uniform materialistic machine that has no free individuality. The body can be seen as the physical-chemical vehicle that carries inherited dispositions from the forefathers, that may transmit inherited defects to certain organs of the body, for instance the limbic-dopamine system of the brain, resulting in an addictive physical disposition. The psyche can be regarded as that independent organisation of psychological functions constituted out of cognitive activities, feeling responses, perceptions and sensations and willed actions, that will create, drive and express the personality in very specific ways to develop, for instance, an addictive personality. The spirit can be seen as an independent free domain of higher truth and goodness, out of which resources can be drawn for learning, growing and healing, where, for instance, new impulses can be taken up by the *I* or *higher Self* of the addict to overcome her dependency.

Within this picture of the body-soul-spirit continuum, it is natural to expect the body, as the vehicle for soul and spirit, to mirror and express the imprint and activity of the soul and spirit within it. There will have to be physical and chemical correlates for every psycho-spiritual activity that takes place within the realm of the body. Thus the different parts of the brain will reflect the activity of the soul and spirit working through it. The addict who is craving a drug as if her survival depended on it, will manifest in the limbic region of the brain dopamine-like neuro-hormones as the chemical correlates for her psychosomatic needs, the expression of those will forces that manifest in her drives or desires.

With this understanding of addiction, and the vulnerability of children and adolescents to getting hooked into this world of dependency, we can now explore a rational and effective way of managing this problem.

Chapter 3. Managing Addictions in Children and Young Adults

Awakening to addiction opens the door to its understanding. Understanding is the journey to effective caring. This journey has been my quest to find an effective way of managing addictions. It requires partnership and participation. It calls for courage and motivation. It needs me to face pain and discomfort. But it will lead to the reclaiming and reordering of a life and a meeting with the true self.

⁓

Effective management of addiction in childhood and adolescence rests on four basic principles: a good understanding of addiction, self-reflection and self-management, understanding the specific child in his specific context and providing a good management plan that can be actively and practically implemented.

Understanding the nature of addiction

We have described in the previous chapter the elements needed for an in-depth understanding of addictions in childhood and youth, and in summary this can be outlined as follows:

- understand needs and gratification;
- understand dependency;
- know the road map of holistic child and adolescent development;
- understand the psychodynamics of addiction.

Addictive behaviour is invariably a cry for help. It is a statement that the child's real inner needs are not being met, forcing him to look elsewhere for his fulfilment. This fundamental understanding is the firm platform upon which other information about the dependent behaviour of the specific child and all future management is based.

Self-reflection and self-care

Before one is in a position to listen openly and objectively to a child in need, one has to clear first one's own inner agenda. This requires one to focus on oneself, checking on one's own inner emotional responses, one's preconceptions and prejudices and doing whatever is needed to clean one's inner screen. Too often we think we are reacting to the child's issues, whereas deeper self-reflection reveals that the reaction has to do with our own unresolved issues which the child simply triggers in us. To gain in-depth understanding of these inner dynamics, and the means to manage them effectively, often requires professional counselling.

Understanding a specific child and his needs

Developmental phase of the child

It is essential right from the start to know clearly where a child is in his developmental journey.

Experiencing the child in his dependency

In Chapter 2 an approach to acquiring a deeper awareness of childhood experience, and in particular of addictive behaviour in children, was described. Having removed one's own personal agenda from the interaction with the child, the focus can now be directed to the child himself whose physical, kinesthetic, thought and ego-profile can be keenly observed.

Next one can identify to a certain degree with the child's experience through conscious empathetic imitation of the child, in the manner of an actor who personifies a particular character.

Finally, one can observe one's portrayal of the child by stepping back and observing the picture one has created in the manner described in the previous chapter. Through self-reflection, one can give added meaning to the experience that the child is going through.

Specific insight into the child's nature: constitution, temperament, character

Apart from having a general plan of the child's development, it is helpful to try to gain some understanding of this specific child's nature. For instance, a melancholic child will respond differently to unfulfilled needs compared to a choleric child.

Thomas is a highly choleric child. His mother will discover that it is never a good idea to lock horns with him when he wants something badly. Choleric children are always right when they are in action or reaction. She realises she can only appeal afterwards to his sense of right and wrong.

Sarah, on the other hand, is a melancholic child. She feels the weight of the world's problems on her fragile shoulders. I can best win her trust when she comes to feel that I understand her troubles, that I have been there and somewhere I suffer with her.

Pandora has a personality that tends to be submissive. His phlegmatic temperament inclines him to want to enjoy his comforts and to avoid as much discomfort as possible. If we are to work effectively with Pandora, we will need to find a way of inspiring and motivating him, by discovering a resource within him that provides him with maximum comfort and support.

It goes beyond the scope of this book to characterise these differences. There is a wealth of literature that offers insight into the constitution, temperament and personality of children and adolescents.[1,2,3]

Insight into the child's environment

It is essential to look at the child within the context of his home, school and social environment.

Sarah lived with her mother, stepfather and their two young children. She experienced herself as the outsider in this home. Her mother was a well-known artist who had very little time for her fifteen-year-old daughter. The pressures of school were heavy and there was no one there who she felt understood her. She found comfort in a small group of rebellious friends who dressed in Gothic outfits and hairdo's, and did all they could to shock the world.

As a young child, Thomas was allowed to watch as much TV as he wished and later a computer was installed in his bedroom. His mother was unhappy in her marriage and his father was often away on business. He was an A grade student who never needed to study to excel at school. He was part of a group of friends who were all obsessed with computer games and would spend hours on the weekends playing these games.

Because there has been no one monitoring his activities, Pandora has been able to do what he likes after school since both parents work the whole day and have little interest in his life. His schoolteachers have not taken a personal interest in him and allowed him to slip behind in his schoolwork. He was at one time very enthusiastic about judo but without encouragement, this, like other social activities, came to an end.

Attitudinal change to the addicted child

When we realise that we all have dependencies of one kind or another and that the child's addiction is an extreme along the life dependency curve, we will have more compassion and understanding for his unfulfilled needs. We will be better able to accept the child without accepting the addictive habit. There is no place for judgment or condemnation, and feelings of parental shame and guilt need to be dealt with. We need to acknowledge that the child has the right to expect that his life needs are provided by his environment. Are we providing what the child needs? Is the child's addiction telling us something about our own obsessive or fixed character? Can we change our attitude to meet these children who are growing up so fast in a world so different from the one in which we grew up?

Assessing the degree of the child's addictive behaviour

It is essential to obtain an accurate idea of the child's addictive nature. Many children go through fads and fashions without getting harmfully addicted. Each addiction will have its own physical, psychological and social expression and will be described comprehensively in the following chapters. However in general one will need to be attentive to a deterioration in physical health, for instance, tiredness, change in eating and sleeping patterns, weight changes, and so on; and a change in psycho-social behaviour, such as withdrawal, irritability, agitation or loss of motivation.

In addition one would like to know the extent and frequency of the addictive habit, for instance, when and how frequently drugs are taken, what is the duration and frequency of TV and computer usage, does the child have access to pornographic websites, and so on? These factors will determine the impact on the child's social, emotional, mental and spiritual development.

Effective management

The key to managing an addictive problem is to *create a partnership* with the dependent person and to achieve this, *effective communication* is needed. Every attempt should be made to engage the child in open and honest conversation about the addictive behaviour. He needs to be challenged to face himself critically and responsibly with initiative and freedom. He also needs to be clearly informed about the nature and dangers of the addictive behaviour. Above all, the conscience and the intuitive knowing of the child needs to be touched. However this will only be possible if the child trusts you. For this he needs to be respected, heard and understood. And this may take as long as is needed for the child to feel safe and trusting.

I am convinced that every adult who has the interests of the child at heart will have the intuitive skill to help the child in need. While some people have a natural way with children, making them feel immediately at ease, all of us can help children *by simply showing interest in them and learning to listen to them.* This begins with providing a good ear and an open heart. We can enhance our skills by applying certain basic rules and conditions in listening and speaking to children.

Conditions for effective communication

- *The child needs to feel safe and accepted before he will speak freely.* This is the first precondition of effective counselling, something that is very often forgotten even by experienced counsellors, wasting time and energy. By establishing safety conditions at the outset, you are signalling to the child that you are on his side. All the things that would make him reluctant to talk, such as fear of consequences, shame at divulging information, fear of rejection, of hurting parents, displeasing them, and so on, must be cleared up before any other work is done.

- *Empathic listening tells the child you are interested in him.* Some people are born with this gift, others have to train themselves to acquire the skill. Listening with an open heart is half the job done. Children know intuitively when an adult is listening to them fully, partially or not at all. A child will feel increased self-esteem the more an adult is interested in him and will naturally open up faster and far more deeply. Empathy can, of itself, be a healing factor that redresses previous ruptures in trust.

- *The child will feel supported if he feels that his talking and sharing is teamwork.* Most children love to work in groups and like to feel they are part of a team, where they are equal, important and a valued partner, carrying the respect and trust that a successful partnership needs. At the same time, the child needs to feel the support of an adult who he feels understands where he is. If the child feels that the adult 'has been there', knows what he is going through, understands, accepts, encourages and supports him, then he can get through almost anything.

Ethical guidelines

If one wishes to connect more deeply with the child in distress there are certain *ethical principles* that make a huge difference in communicating with or counselling children. For even when the child is trapped in addictive behaviour, the innate trust in the child's potential can become the highest ethical standards out of which wisdom and healing can flow to children in distress. The ethical principles used in the psychophonetic counselling process form the cornerstone of these guidelines.[4]

In his full being, the child is inwardly equipped for the journey of his life

He has the inner wisdom, strength, resilience and resources needed and he will know intuitively the next step, if we allow him the freedom to express it. Very often the child cannot articulate this wisdom and needs the adult to do this for him. We need to provide options for the child; our words may then strike his soul like a bell in order for his own wisdom to resonate from him. The assumption is commonly to regard children as inexperienced, helpless, weak and unable to take responsibility for their lives. The caregiver will then consciously or unconsciously take over the problem from his point of reference, thereby disempowering the child in his necessary learning experience. This violates the enshrined principle to respect and trust the child's inner resources. On the other hand, adult expectations can be placed on the child, projecting on him capacities that he has not yet acquired. He may then feel out of his depth and completely unsupported.

The child, in his unborn nature, carries the innate guidance for his own life journey

This arises out of the power of will that is the very essence of the human *I* of the child. As we have seen, instincts, drives, desires, motivation, wishes, intentions, resolutions and actions are part of this inner guidance. Every crisis or difficulty in which the child finds himself is a learning and a growing opportunity and the child's authority with regard to his own growing process should be completely respected. Our wise counsel should be carefully and tentatively offered to the child out of the feeling-knowing resonances that the child is allowed to bring forward himself. There is always the temptation, as the knowing, caring and responsible adult, to take charge of the process and to give advice that may well be right for the carer but completely off the mark for the child. Many children will choose not to speak about their problems even to the most trusting adult because they are not yet ready to do so. We should respect the child's freedom to be silent and to choose with whom and when they wish to speak; they well know the reasons why they need to be silent.

The child, as the author of his experience, will create his own meaning out of this experience

Respecting the child means trusting that what a child experiences is real and that the meaning he gives it is to be fully respected. This meaning needs to be unconditionally heard and validated and requires to be kept apart from any other viewpoints, past events or future action. The meaning that the child gives to his experience has its integral truth and reality.

The child is always in the process of rhythmical incarnation and development

This means that his nature is always changing and if we are to gain his trust we need to know where he is in his process of development. Every age requires a different approach. It is completely different talking to a child of seven years, to one of nine, thirteen, fifteen or seventeen.

The child is preparing for the birth of his I nature

This takes place in the twentieth year of life. Until then, the I is imprinting itself step by step into the psychosomatic life of the developing child. The I is not yet free of its other organic and psychological responsibilities to be able to invest in pure spiritual activities, and therefore needs to be protected by the developed I of an adult. Like the picture of Christopherus carrying his tiny but mighty child on his shoulders through a strong flowing river (Figure 2), so the protective power of the adult I should look after the budding life and power of the child's being with love, care and deep respect.

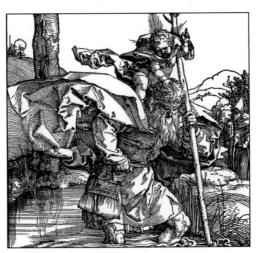

Figure 2. Albrecht Dürer, St Christopher.

Once a partnership based on trust and mutual respect has been established, there are a number of other factors that are critical for an effective management programme:

Motivation, commitment, contracts, accountability and realistic time frames

Team effort

Where possible the therapeutic team (doctor, counsellor, therapist), which obviously includes the client, needs to be working together with family members, school teachers and other community-based adults who interact with the child in sport clubs, religious or other associations. The engagement of the members of this team in the rehabilitation process needs to be negotiated with the child himself, for he needs to have a say in their involvement in his healing. Once he has overcome his shame and mistrust and he has agreed to work together with selected personnel, the child or youth will gain confidence to have members of his close community involved in his programme.

Trust and the feeling of support will lead to self-motivation to engage actively in managing the problem. If there is sufficient enthusiasm and motivation, the client will be more inclined to make commitments, which should be structured into a contract signed by all parties concerned. The client should hold himself accountable in ways that are negotiated and that can be practically applied. Short-term rather than long-term time frames should be set down, with regular opportunity for monitoring and review.

The stage is now set for the construction of an individual therapeutic programme.

Clinical, therapeutic and detox management

These programmes will differ according to the specific clinical orientation of the health practitioners involved. The programme offered by the Syringa Integrated Health Centre in Cape Town, where I work, integrates conventional and complementary medical interventions into an holistic approach. This includes:

- individual dietary and nutritional interventions;
- detox programmes using oral and intravenous procedures;
- individually-prescribed neutraceutical, herbal and homeopathic medication;
- a range of therapeutic options such as rhythmical massage, art therapy, eurythmy therapy, speech therapy;
- equine-assisted therapy (hippotherapy);
- counselling.[5]

Counselling

This is an essential part of the therapeutic programme. Psychophonetics is the counselling approach that has proven to be most effective in my work with addictions. Working with children requires a completely different counselling approach to working with adults, because of their developmental process and the fact that they have not yet awakened to their *I* nature. This is why parents or guardians need to be actively involved in the counselling process and indeed for children before puberty, a guardian needs *always* to be present with the child being counselled.

Counselling children in different life phases

Each life phase of the child requires a different counselling approach.

As described in the previous chapter, a child younger than seven years is working on his own biological organisation and therefore still lives within and depends on the life sheath of his parents. This life sheath represents the mature biological functions of those adults who nurture and care for him. It sustains him and provides him with his basic biological needs. His soul life, too, is still bound up with this biological development and therefore is not freely available for an independent engagement with the counsellor. The counsellor needs to be aware of the biological life environment of the child and will engage with the child from within this sphere. Counsellors need to be conscious of their own biological functions, for instance their energy and breathing functions, which will affect the young child.

Between seven and fourteen years, a part of the soul life begins to awaken from its slumber within the body. The feelings begin to free themselves from their biological attachment and the child begins his agonising and ecstatic journey into new inner experiences. During this period his delicate soul life is embraced and protected by the soul sheath of parents, carers and teachers, whose matured and awakened soul life can hold the growing soul as it gradually emerges, free and vulnerable, into the outer world. It is into this sheath that we as counsellors must enter with the greatest reverence, knowing that our psyche will have a direct effect on his developing soul.

Puberty heralds the birth of the soul life. As the faculty of rational and independent thinking takes on a life of its own, the will, driven by the reproductive and hormonal system, drives the youth into new and powerful worldly experiences. The soul awakens fresh and curious to discover the world in a new and independent way. Being so open and awake, it is highly sensitive to these unfiltered impressions and needs to be protected by the *I* sheath of adults in his community. These are adults whose own *I* natures are mature and integrated enough to respectfully be present for the youth as he is growing towards the birth of his own *I* in his twentieth year. As counsellors we shall need to be active within this *I* sheath of the adolescent client, offering for him a role model for that to which he aspires.

Fundamental elements in psychophonetic counselling of addictions

There are several essential elements that are fundamental to the psychophonetic counselling approach of addictions:

- The exploration and discovery in a safe environment of *real unfulfilled suppressed needs,* leading to the adoption of the substitutive dependency response.

In our initial conversation Sarah found the safety, trust and courage to begin the counselling process. The first step was to discover the hidden suppressed needy person who was desperate to be seen, heard and understood. The lack of this acknowledgment in her life was the source of her deep hurt. Sarah quickly understood why she became dependent on cutting as a way of drawing attention to herself.

- The facing and exposing of the *hostile nature* of the substitutive dependency response.

The next step for Sarah was to face the activity of cutting as an entity that helped her gain exposure and attention. She had to enter into it as if she was playing the character of the 'cutter'. When she looked at the after-image of herself as the 'cutter' she was horrified to discover a powerful adult woman who experienced pleasure in cutting a young child, allowing the inner child to feel wanted and relevant. She named this 'cutter' part of herself as the 'paedophile'.

- The finding of new, creative, healthy, real inner resources for addressing these underlying needs.

Sarah could see that she needed the loving care of an attentive mother who would take time to listen to her and to understand her. She was sure that her biological mother would never be able to give her this. Besides, she did not want this from her own mother. She resolved to find this within herself. She knew exactly what she wanted and called up this imagined experience as if she was playing the part of a warm loving mother. In this role she was able to connect deeply with the needy child, initiating a new relationship that could effectively address her unfulfilled need. She also decisively removed the child from the clutches of the paedophile.

- The energetic and consistent implementation in life of these new found resources as a powerful alternative to the addictive habit.

Although this counselling work in itself gave Sarah the impetus to stop cutting, it was important that Sarah continued in her own time, over the following weeks, to enact the different roles and their interaction, so as to consolidate the new intervention and to consciously counteract the old addictive habit. For as long as a primary need is still unfulfilled, it will look elsewhere for its gratification.

In the chapters ahead, the specific case studies will illustrate the way in which psychophonetic counselling works in the different types of addictions.

Referral to specialist care and rehab centres

In cases where there is no motivation to change, in uncontrolled addiction and in devious addictive behaviour, referral to psychiatrists, psychologists and admission to clinics and rehabilitation centres may be unavoidable. The child or youth in such cases needs to be protected from his own destructive nature and may require containing medication, hospitalisation or referral to centres that offer in-house care and rehabilitative support

The challenge and opportunity of addiction

The challenge of addiction is the struggle for freedom from entrapment and dependency.

—

As was said before, one of the greatest tasks facing every human being is the ongoing struggle between the egoistic needs of the soul and the higher non-selfish aspirations of the spirit. The former tie one down to personal and egoistic inclinations and antipathies; the latter open one up to more global opportunities that serve more than just the personal self. This is not to say that the needs of the body and soul are not of great value to the human being; for the child is a being of body whose biological needs have to be served, and also a being of soul whose psychological needs seek to be gratified.

The soul stands between body and spirit. This means that there is a part of the soul that will serve the bodily needs; the desire and liking for food will support the physiological requirements of the body. There is also a part of the soul that will serve the aspirations of the spirit; thinking capacities will create a clear path to fulfilling the ideals of the higher self.

In every human being there is a great longing to unfold and express his higher self. That is perhaps why every person is striving to become something, to improve himself and to discover what gives him the greatest joy, peace and fulfilment. He will go to extraordinary ends to find this and will overcome the greatest obstacles to achieve it.

Addiction has been present as a condition of the soul from time immemorial. In our age, it has become a very powerful, challenging force. It has the power to subordinate the self and cripple the destinies of many children and adolescents, preventing them from discovering their true potential. Or, it can offer the opportunity for the self to overcome a great obstacle and through this victory discover the great power for good that is alive within the self.

Chapter 4. Food Addictions and Disorders

I experience food as something warming and comforting, like a kind and loving mother that provides nurture and care for my bodily needs. I am intrigued to explore why children with food and eating addictions use food or the lack of it to appease unfulfilled needs. What lives behind their disturbed relationship with food or eating?

—

Many children use food to appease the inner pain of real needs that are not addressed. They discover that food in general, specific foods, large quantities or tiny amounts may provide brief or sustained respite, pleasure or protection from their inner discomforts.

A variety of well-documented eating disorders in children and adolescents can all be regarded as outcomes of food-related addiction. We shall examine the eating disorders of young children as well as those in older children and adolescents. Common to them all are unhealthy eating habits that are used as a means of coping with psychological discomforts such as boredom, frustration, abandonment, insecurity, fear, loneliness, unhappiness and rejection. They are repetitive patterns of behaviour using food, or the lack of it, to satisfy deeper real needs that are not met.

It is also common to find unresolved traumas of children in food substance addiction.

Eating disorders in young children

Pica

Two year old Samantha has a habit of licking the walls in her bedroom and often eats sand from the flower pot. Her mother was fifteen years old when she gave birth to Samantha who was given to foster care parents, both of whom were working people and were out most of the day.

Pica is a condition where infants persistently eat non-nutritive substances such as hair, cloth, paint, lime wash or plaster, and older children eat pebbles, sand, animal faeces, insects, flowers, leaves, and so on. It usually occurs in the second or third year of life. Pica may occur in autistic and mentally-impaired children. More often it is due to a specific nutritional deficiency such as calcium, iron or zinc. It may also be due to a neglectful or otherwise deficient mother-child relationship. In both situations, there is the instinctive attempt to replace either biologically or psychologically what is missing. Pica may be a risk factor for uncontrolled eating behaviour in adolescence.[1]

Food refusal and pickiness

Shanti was never a good feeder as an infant; she suffered from post-natal colic and reflux and was later diagnosed as lactose intolerant. As a young child she was a fussy eater, refusing many foods and always picking on her food. She was a nervous and highly strung child; her anxious mother and aggressive father divorced when she was two years old and they continued for years to be argumentative and reactive whenever they saw each other.

This is a very common occurrence in children of all ages and has various causes. In toddlers and early schoolchildren, feeding problems and eating disturbances occur in 25–40% of the population.[2] In most cases it is a transient behavioural problem and not a serious threat to health. In older pre-pubertal children there is uncertainty whether this represents an earlier version of anorexia nervosa, yet the health risks may be just as serious as those for older girls with a clear diagnosis. Functional digestive disturbances and food sensitivities cause digestive discomfort and resistance to eating. The parental-child relationship, especially regarding food and mealtimes, plays a major role in refusing food. Some parents are misguided about what constitutes a healthy diet and impose rigid controls or anxiety-charged expectations on sensitive children. There may be no regular mealtimes when parents and children sit together; a mother may force-feed her child or demand that all food on the plate be finished; the mother who is over stressed, diet and weight conscious and irritable at mealtimes, imparts to the child an anxiety which she associates with eating. It is very frequently the mother-child relationship which is at the root of the problem, leading to unsatisfied oral needs of the child. Although this is a very common occurrence that cannot be regarded as addictive behaviour, it appears likely that in predisposed children, this pattern of behaviour can set the stage for more serious food dependency problems later on. Some researchers believe that food refusal, pickiness and digestive problems are risk factors for subsequent anorexia, but this is contested by other research.[3]

Overweight and obesity

Four-year-old Precious is ten kilos (22 lb) overweight. Although she was not a big baby, she was never breastfed and was reared on a fortified formula feed. She lives with her mother and six other children in an informal settlement outside Cape Town. Her mother is obese and has fed the family largely on a diet of corn and beans.

Obese and overweight infants and toddlers are an everyday sight and the number has tripled in the last thirty years. Approximately 10% of children aged two to five years are overweight. Obesity in early life is characterised by increased number and size of fat cells. Once this has been established, it is physiologically difficult to change and predisposes to adult obesity. A preschool obese child has a 30–40% chance of becoming an obese adult.[4] The tendency to put on weight may be genetic in origin (see below) or diet related. Overfeeding of infants in the first year of life tends to occur more with artificial feeding as opposed to breastfeeding; mothers tend to encourage infants to finish the bottle and the baby is unable to control milk intake to the same extent as is possible on the breast. However, psychological factors are invariably also implicated: for instance, a mother who cannot bond with her child, who is overanxious or has misconceptions about food will tend to overfeed her child. These children are prone to repeated respiratory and gastro-intestinal infections and their impaired sugar metabolism predisposes them to sugar diabetes.

Eating disorders in older children and adolescents

Jane contracted rheumatic fever when she was six years old and had to stay in bed for weeks. She felt miserable and bored and she consoled herself by eating throughout the day. When she finally could get out of bed she had put on ten kilos (22 lb) in weight. Her mother was horrified at her appearance, told her how terrible she looked and urged her to stop over-eating. She was teased at school for being fat. She carried deep feelings of inadequacy and self-loathing. She could not stop eating and at the age of thirteen years she was 25 kilos (55 lb) overweight.

Overweight and obesity

Obesity and overweightness has become a global epidemic. Worldwide, at least 10% of school age children are overweight or obese, with the highest prevalence occurring in the Americas (32%), then Europe (20%), and the Middle East (16%). In the USA 40–50% of school age children are overweight and approximately 15–18% are obese. In the UK, 30–40% of teenagers are overweight, while 15–20% are obese.[5,6,7] This is a worldwide phenomenon occurring in both developed and most developing countries, although the increase is seen more dramatically in economically developed countries and in urbanised populations.

Obesity is defined as excessive fat accumulation in the body that causes the body weight to exceed 20% of the standard weight as determined by height and weight tables. Overweight is a 10% excess of the desired weight.

Increase in body weight seems to be determined by an interaction between genetic, environmental and psycho-social factors, leading to a greater intake of calories or energy than can be expended.

Several genes have been associated with human obesity and its metabolic complications and although no specific genetic marker has been identified, it seems likely that multiple genes acting in combination influence the biochemical pathways involved in the complex neuro-endocrine control of hunger and food intake. In animals, selective breeding can easily produce increased fat, suggesting that genetics play a part in fat production. Eighty percent of obese people have a family history of obesity, and identical twins raised apart can both be obese.

The environmental factor can be seen in the higher prevalence of

63

obesity in industrialised countries, both among lower socio-economic sections as well as more affluent sectors, in unhealthy eating and in lack of exercise. In preschool and school years, obesity is promoted by the excessive intake of food, especially highly refined carbohydrates such as sugar, sweetened drinks, white bread, cakes and sweets, and high fat diets such as butter, fried foods and fatty meat. Fat, moreover, has a weak ability to satisfy appetite. The regular consumption of fast foods, sweetened drinks and even fruit juices will also promote obesity. Research indicates that children who eat lunch at school food shops are at increased risk of gaining weight; those who eat supper with their family three or more times a week are at decreased risk, and kids in high income neighbourhoods were half as likely to become overweight than their peers in low income areas. Decrease in physical activity restricts energy consumption and may contribute to increased food intake. In developed countries a clear relationship exists between low levels of physical activity and obesity. There is also a clear association between TV hours and obesity.

Psycho-social factors play a central role. Children learn to use overeating as a means of coping with their psycho-emotional problems. Parental and peer attitudes to the overweight child, as well as parental overweightness, appear to be potent factors in obesity.

Excessive weight in children should be regarded as a serious disease which predisposes the child to a wide range of health problems: physical discomfort, the overtaxing of many organ systems, skeletal complications (for instance, flat feet) and the rising incidence of juvenile diabetes are some of the physical consequences. Feelings of low self-esteem and poor self-image, intensified by the social consequences of poor school performance, discrimination and loss of friends, lead to self-loathing and depression, all of which perpetuate the addictive eating tendency.

Children who were heavy babies at birth, or children who become obese, have a much greater chance of growing into obese adults who are at great risk of developing some of the most prevalent and life-threatening diseases of modern society. These include sugar diabetes, cardiovascular disease, high blood pressure, raised cholesterol, gallstones and cancer.

Sugar craving

Sugar and sugar products are well known as comfort or reward foods. What is your relationship to sweet food? Many of us feel nurtured, rewarded and comforted by sweet foods and many young people will crave sugar-rich foods to try to relieve feelings of inner discomfort. Is this experience familiar to you? Sugar is the prime source of short term energy. When our blood sugar drops we feel tired and weak; we take sugar and we feel energised again. Children unconsciously sense the power that sugar gives them and those who constitutionally lack energy and drive will tend to crave for sweet foods. Sugar products are often given to children as a treat, reward or bribe to make them feel better or to get them to behave better. They learn that sugar is a special reward food which gives pleasure and creates a happier, more likeable person. It is therefore not very difficult for children to develop an addiction for sweet foods.

Today the average person in the USA and UK consumes her weight in sugar in one year. A 2011 survey of 2,157 teenagers aged twelve to eighteen years found the average daily consumption of added sugars was 119 grams (4 oz) or 28.3 teaspoons![8] Many children in all socio-economic strata have replaced drinking water with sweetened drinks or fruit juices. Almost all overweight and obese children consume vast amounts of sugar daily which is undoubtedly leading to the huge surge in adult type diabetes at an increasingly younger age.

The constant dumping of sugar into the liver will weaken this organ, causing an increased tendency to allergies and recurrent infections. Sugar laden party foods are probably the major factor causing recurrent upper respiratory infections that ultimately lead to removal of tonsils, adenoids and the insertion of grommets. These childhood operations are frequently found later in the medical history of patients with digestive and liver disturbances. Other children are highly sensitive to sugar, contributing to conditions like Attention Deficit Disorder, with or without hyperactivity and learning difficulties.

Controlled eating and anorexia nervosa

Ayesha was a timid, diligent and conventional sixteen-year-old girl who was always a fussy eater. Her mother herself was diet and weight conscious and extremely protective and caring of her daughter. Ayesha carried huge anxiety about life, about herself, forming relationships, and having children. Her parents started noticing her greater preoccupation with food and with it, her failure to gain weight. She started exercising compulsively, refusing food and dropped her weight critically. She felt safe in the choices she had made for herself.

Abnormal eating habits leading to controlled eating and weight loss, with its extreme form in anorexia nervosa, is widespread in all developed countries. Anorexia is much more prevalent in western culture but seems to be on the rise in non-western countries. In South Africa it is increasing among of all racial groups who follow a developing western culture. A preliminary study in secondary school girls in South Africa suggests that one in five girls has abnormal eating attitudes and up to 5% of young women will exhibit some of the symptoms of anorexia.[9]

This tendency usually manifests in the mid-teens, but may appear any time between ten and thirty years of age. Adolescent girls between 17 amd 18 years are most at risk. It occurs ten to twenty times more often in females than in males, with the greatest frequency in professions and competitive activities that require thinness such as modelling, ballet, gymnastics and athletics (1–5% of all female adolescents and young women). It is often associated with a past history of physical or sexual abuse, and with parents who themselves have eating disorders or weight problems.

Anorexia nervosa is characterised by compulsive weight loss due to a morbid fear of gaining weight, together with a misperception of their body weight and shape. There is usually a preoccupation with food and dieting, weight control and body shape, a denial of the seriousness of the problem and a restless pursuit of thinness, often to starvation and even death from multiple organ failure. They usually refuse to eat with their families or in public places, abuse laxatives and diuretics to lose weight and engage in compulsive exercising. They are usually anaemic, feel the cold intensely, often have low energy, feel dizzy or faint easily, are usually constipated and girls typically stop menstruating. Their growth may be stunted in puberty and they may develop osteoporosis later in life. They are moody, depressed and even suicidal. The cause, once again, seems likely to involve many different factors.

The desire to lose weight almost always has a *psycho-emotional* basis. There may be a strong need to take control of some part of her life – her weight, her body image, or body functions such as eating, digesting and menstruating; she may have a subconscious aversion to growing up, preferring a child-like body to the challenges that come with an adult body. She may also find that starving herself produces a euphoric feeling of disconnection from the world, similar to the 'high' experienced from some drugs.

Anorexia occurs predominately in individuals with low self-esteem who are rigid, perfectionist, obsessive and compulsive in nature. They are often shy, studious and over-compliant, and typically lack a sense of autonomy and selfhood and are often unable to separate psychologically from an over-caring mother. Twin studies suggest that genetic/biological factors may predispose to the condition.[10,11] It is still unclear whether associated changes in neurotransmitters and hormones are causes or effects of anorexia.

Socio-cultural factors also play an important role: anorexia nervosa appears to be more common in industrialised nations and is supported by society's emphasis on thinness and exercise that the media equates with personal happiness, love and financial success.

Anorexic girls may be more influenced by advertising and media pressure that encourages slimming, than non-anorexic girls of the same age.[12]

Bulimia nervosa

Roxanne led a secret double life. To outsiders she appeared a normal healthy and popular fifteen-year-old schoolgirl; on the inside she was tormented by obsessions with food and her weight. She would, in public, control her eating habits; secretly she would stuff herself full of foods that gave her transient pleasure; then followed the acute disgust, guilt and remorse and she would resort to vomiting and laxatives to prevent herself gaining weight. She would often cut herself as punishment and had begun to flirt provocatively with boys. Her mother was in an abusive relationship with a gay partner and was herself over-preoccupied with her figure and fashions.

This condition is characterised by recurrent episodes of uncontrolled binge eating combined with inappropriate ways of preventing weight gain such as self-induced vomiting, misuse of laxatives, diuretics, enemas, fasting or excessive exercise. It is more prevalent than anorexia nervosa, occurring in 1–3% of young women, most commonly in late adolescence. As in anorexia nervosa, bulimic patients are over concerned about their body shape and weight and find it extremely difficult to be objective about it. However, unlike anorexia they may maintain a normal body weight. Their health risks are mainly due to the consequences of purging and laxative abuse, and include salivary gland swelling (characteristic chipmunk face), dental enamel erosion, dehydration, tears of the stomach lining, bleeding and even sudden death.

Genetic factors appear to be less important, but low serotonin may play a part in the uncontrolled appetite. They are also subject to the socio-cultural pressures to be slim but their psychological profile is different. They seem to lie somewhere between the extremes of anorexia and obesity: they try to gain self-control by restricting their eating but then completely lose control by secret food binging; this may be followed by purging, with subsequent shame, guilt feelings, depression and suicide. Their lack of self-control makes them generally more outgoing and impulsive, leading them frequently into substance dependence, shoplifting, promiscuity and self-destructive sexual relationships. Their emotional ability allows them to feel and express their anger, frustration, guilt and self disgust.

A preliminary study to determine factors influencing eating attitudes in high school girls in South Africa confirmed other findings that *maternal influences* played an important role in these attitudes: for instance, communications concerning their daughter's weight, food and dieting to lose or gain weight.[13]

Mothers of bulimic daughters more often perceived their daughters to be overweight and encouraged dieting and exercise more than mothers of non-bullimic daughters.[14]

Mothers of adolescents with eating disorders tend themselves to be more prone to eating disorders than mothers of adolescents without eating disorders.[15]

Understanding the nature of food addiction

While the environment provides outer trigger factors, and heredity enhances the predisposition, the constitution of the human being as a continuum of body, soul and spirit must be regarded as the focus for understanding eating disorders. We shall need to explore the human element, in particular find out what is going on within the psyche of the child and examine how this impacts on her body and spirit. As said before, there is no better way than to start with one's own experience.

To begin, we have to first clear our own preconceptions and personal issues about food and eating disorders in order that we can understand the nature of addiction and find genuine interest and respect for the child with a food addiction. How do you feel about eating disorders, addictive tendencies, and the possibility that this child may have an eating addiction? What emotional responses arise in you when these issues confront you? Before one can be attentive and objective towards the child, these issues need first to be acknowledged, addressed and put aside.

This was extremely difficult for someone like Ayesha's mother who herself was still struggling with a similar problem. She had to confront her own issues as the first step towards helping her daughter.

Ayesha's mother consulted me about her daughter's anorexia. She described how fastidious she herself had always been with food and how she had tried her best to bring her children up on the healthiest diet. She admitted she was quite obsessed with health and had fears about many illnesses, especially cancer which had taken the life of her mother when she was still a child. The picture emerged of a highly anxious person whose way of controlling her fears was to control her diet as a way of maintaining her health. She could see how this compulsive behaviour was impacting negatively on her life as well as that of her daughter's. She realised she would have to find the strength to overcome her fear of ill health so that she could let go of the compulsive need to control her diet and health.

Once we have cleared our own inner emotional responses we can turn our attention to the child and try to understand all we can about her, in the methodology described in Chapter 2.

We will begin to realise that Ayesha is carrying a great deal of anxiety and by controlling her eating, she has found a way of controlling her anxiety.

By entering into the inner experience of the children described above, we discover that Samantha, Precious, Jane, Ayesha, and Roxanne are all needy children who have found in food a substitute that gives them regular comfort and satisfaction because their current emotional needs are not being fulfilled. These children all have highly sensitive and vulnerable dispositions; they feel anxious, insecure and unsafe. We can follow the inner biography of each particular child as we did with Pandora and realise that this unfulfilled real need causes the child deep inner discomfort which forces her to search for another substitute which gratifies her need. In each case, food or other ingested substances in one form or another or a particular eating behaviour becomes the false substitute that eases the discomfort for a short while.

Ayesha refuses to eat because of the inner anxiety created in her by her anxious mother. She discovers that by not eating, she feels more in control and her anxiety lessens allowing her to cope better with her anxious mother. Jane, who learnt that eating soothed her boredom, frustration and hurt when she had rheumatic fever, eats compulsively when she feels pressurised by her parents or by her own inadequacies and unworthiness.

In the more severe forms, eating or not eating becomes an habitual means of blocking out emotional pain and discomfort in the same way as a painkiller or sedative is continuously needed to subdue pain or anxiety (see box).

Unfulfilled primary need → pain → blocking of the need → ensuing discomfort → the finding and adopting of a substitute gratification → appeases the pain briefly → secondary need → dependency on substitute agency

---

Food and the maternal stream

The next intriguing question is to ask why these sensitive children choose specifically food to soothe their soul discomfort. Since the *activity of eating* and the *nutritional process* is common to them all, it may be helpful to explore what these processes represent for the growing child.

Food maintains and nurtures the body. The drive for food is one of the basic needs that the soul requires for preservation of the body; young and old, we all feel physically and emotionally satisfied after a good meal, especially one prepared by a caring person, or a loving mother. There appears to be an innate connection between food, eating and maternal nurturing. The nutritional stream nurtures the child physically in the same way as the mother nurtures the child emotionally. One of the earliest associations a newborn baby has with her mother is the warm flow of milk that nourishes her body. The child feels with the inflow of food into her body something similar to the nurturing she receives from her mother. When this psycho-organic need has been fulfilled, the child will feel whole and complete. On a soul level, one may say she tastes the mother; she has a feeling of wellbeing similar to that which she experiences when she rests in the loving arms of her mother or when she feels her mother is there for her. And when her mother is not there or is too much there for her, she may seek food to satisfy her need. Or she may reject food.[16]

Food addictions may well express some dysfunction between the child, its body and the stream of nurturing with which the maternal energy is intimately connected. Research in this field seems to indicate that the mother plays a crucial role in eating disorders: this is evident in the early eating disorders of food refusal, pica and overweight. Children who overeat may be expressing the longing for the mother or the wish to identify with the mother who represents for them the protection and nurturing that they are not yet able to give themselves. Anorexia nervosa is often associated with a mother who was frequently absent, smothering or too controlling, or a distorted relationship with a father, which disturbs the maternal connection. These children may be making a conscious or unconscious attempt to distance themselves from the maternal stream and to establish their own autonomy. They seem to have an aversion for everything that connects their body with the mother or womanhood: their menstruation, sexuality, relationships and eating. They take on a more masculine and cerebral persona; they seem to disconnect from life and become more spiritual; in contrast the obese child has a more feminine and heartfelt nature; they hide behind an expanded body and become more earthly. Adolescents who overeat and then purge themselves may be expressing the struggle for separation from a maternal figure who they alternately wish to hold on to (overeating) and then wish to free themselves from (purging). Many girls with eating disorders have a history of sexual abuse.[17]

The eating disorders of older children manifest at a time when the child is faced with powerful developmental challenges – physically, emotionally and socially. Puberty awakens the child to the vulnerability of body and soul; adolescence is characterised by the striving for a sense of identity and a new sense of self; there are healthy and less healthy responses to these challenges. These food addictions and eating disorders may be an attempt to provide protection, autonomy and self-definition in the face of these developmental challenges.

Helping youngsters with food addictions

Prevention is always better than cure. Parents and especially mothers – the usual food providers – need to be well guided in all aspects relating to food and eating. The following are some guidelines that will reduce the incidence of eating disorders:

- Exclusive breastfeeding for at least six months should be encouraged, especially for mothers who have a family history of obesity.
- Acquire a clear understanding of the quality and quantity of a healthy balanced diet for each appropriate age, from an expert in the field. Avoid unnecessary refined foods, fat and sugar products. Parents should demonstrate balance in eating; all foods can be enjoyed in moderation. Do not label food good or bad.
- Provide quality time for meals with children, free of anxiety or disharmony.
- Exercise should be balanced, recreational and fun for children; exercise used competitively and to lose weight is harmful for young children.
- Examine your own attitudes towards eating and body image, especially mothers who serve as role models for daughters. The mother's perception of physical appearances can and often does have a profound effect on a child's belief system and actions. This is also important for fathers because their views of women profoundly affect their daughters' self-image and understanding of what the opposite sex will expect of them.
- One of the most important times to identify and prevent potential obesity is at the age of 12–18 months, since being overweight at this age seems to be an indicator for obesity in later life.
- Children with poor or fussy appetites should be carefully monitored without drawing attention to their food. Medical conditions that cause loss of appetite obviously need to be excluded. Explore possible causes with an informed practitioner and find creative ways of encouraging eating. Using food as a punishment or reward is usually not effective, and may be harmful.

Sensitive management of children with food addictions and eating disorders can make a huge difference to outcomes, and the approach outlined in the previous chapter is designed to understand the child maximally and provide her with optimum care and support.

The preliminary steps require that firstly we are there for the child and not distracted by our own personal issues; secondly that we know something about the nature of addiction; and thirdly that we have taken the trouble to try to understand the child in the way described above.

We use all our senses to observe the child as keenly as possible gaining a comprehensive picture of her physical, kinaesthetic and psychological profile. We consider what kind of temperament and character she has and in what kind of environment she is living. We try to assess as accurately as possible the degree of her addictive behaviour. Do we know how much she eats, when she eats, where she eats? Do we know about her exercise patterns? Is she using diuretics or laxatives, does she resort to vomiting up her food? What is her health status like and is there any change in behaviour patterns?

It is important to try to detect the warning signs of eating disorders as early as possible, as this may prevent serious developments and minimise the long term damage. Look out for signs of persistent weight gain or sudden weight loss, preoccupation with food and dieting, restrictive eating patterns or evidence of binge eating, unusual or ritualised eating habits, excessive exercising, loss of menstruation, dry sallow skin, hair loss and fine hair growth; bathroom breaks during or after meals suggest vomiting; chipmunk cheeks which are a sign of excess vomiting; baggy or full-cover clothes which are an attempt to hide thinness. These physical signs may be accompanied by mood and behaviour changes such as loss of self-esteem, withdrawal from family and friends, obsessive compulsive behaviour, fear of being overweight and weight loss denial, anxiety, depression and reactive behaviour.

At the same time we carry in the background of our minds an awareness of the road map of development, placing this child in a specific life phase with all its imperatives that will determine her individual needs and their gratification.

We may enter more deeply into the inner experience of the child by conscious empathetic imitation. Deep respectful listening in this manner will usually reveal that these are highly sensitive and vulnerable children and that their eating response, although not healthy, is the best defence they have at their disposal. By acknowledging and accepting their reality as their true experience, and supporting them in their deepest vulnerability, we will gain their trust and establish an effective working partnership. The best communication is one that honours and respects these children's experience, paying heed to those principles and guidelines described in Chapter 3. In this way we will swiftly find out what their real needs are and what they are really missing.

Each specific eating disorder will require an individual programme of management and will differ according to specialist bias and expertise.[18]

The child will first need careful clinical and diagnostic assessment. On this basis, a therapeutic programme will be designed. This will include dietary and nutritional interventions, individually prescribed natural medication, and a range of therapeutic options such as rhythmical massage, craniosacral therapy, art therapy, movement therapy such as eurythmy therapy, hippotherapy and most importantly, counselling, both for family members and the affected child. In severe cases, referral to specialist care and clinical admissions may be required.

Psychophonetic counselling is well suited for children with eating disorders. Its use of verbal as well as non-verbal expressive approaches allow the child to directly discover her vulnerability and what she is missing, as well as new resources to provide for herself the protection and nurturing she needs.

Ayesha was able to verbalise and role-play her vulnerable nature, finding there a highly anxious child, frightened of being alone and feeling very unsafe without the support of her mother. She discovered she was missing deep maternal caring and had to call up within herself this very quality and make it available for her anxious nature. By practising these different aspects of herself, she found within a few weeks that she was far less anxious, far less needy and therefore had less and less desire to exercise rigid control over her eating and exercise activities. Within a few months she had overcome her obsessive and addictive tendencies.

Food addictions and eating disorders are an attempt by some sensitive children to cope with their internal struggles and their life challenges; the use of their bodies and the nutritional process may be an attempt to come to terms with maternal relationships and the mother or woman-nature within themselves; understanding their needs may help us to steer them into safer and healthier directions.

Chapter 5. Sanctioned Substance Abuse

When I look around and observe the habits of people and their social customs, I see the common use of highly addictive substances in everyday life. Their common usage and free availability make it inevitable that young children and youth will partake of them. I wish to understand these drugs that society has so unconditionally embraced, drugs that put the health of so many of our children in danger. I wish to find the right way to deal with these drugs that may devastate the life of a child.

—

There are three drugs that have become so fully integrated into the customs and traditions of societies all over the world that they are hardly regarded as drugs, and yet they have highly addictive potential. These are *caffeine, nicotine* and *ethanol.*

What is your experience of these drugs?

Coffee in the morning, smoking several cigarettes in the day and an alcoholic drink in the evening is a routine part of many people's lives. How do you regard these substances? Do you consider them like food or drink that sustains the body? Are you aware that they are drugs that have a particular physiological effect? Do you notice that they satisfy a particular need beyond the appeasing of hunger or thirst?

It may be instructive to recall your experience and the effects that these three substances have had on you in the past.

What is a drug?

A drug may be defined as a chemical substance having a well defined pharmacological action intended for use in the medical diagnosis, cure, treatment, or prevention of disease. This means that, unlike food substances, they create a predictable change in function such as increased heart rate or change in blood flow. A further definition refers to those substances upon which a person may become dependent or develop tolerance.[1] This means that it becomes difficult to stop the drug without unpleasant withdrawal effects occurring and that after a period of time, one develops a tolerance to the same amount of drug and more is needed to produce the same effects.

These three drugs are present in their natural form as coffee and tea, tobacco and alcohol. When their active ingredients are pharmacologically isolated these are declared scheduled substances and only available on doctor's prescription. Yet in their natural state, and when placed into beverages such as Coca Cola, Red Bull or coffee, they are not subject to any controls or, in the case of nicotine and alcohol, are subject to age restrictions which are very easily circumvented. In reality they are freely available, widely sanctioned and promoted actively by commercial interests.

These substances have become socially acceptable drugs because of the important role they play in enhancing social interaction. They do this in a variety of ways: they facilitate communication by reducing inhibitions and promoting social awareness and wellbeing; they create pleasure and enjoyment through their physical and psychological effects as well as through creating social fusion; and in some cases they enhance efficiency and performance. In most situations their effects are innocuous to the user and advantageous to the social interaction. However, due to their addictive nature, they have the potential to be abused and cause dependency like any other dependency creating substance.

Because caffeine, tobacco and alcohol are so easily accessible, teens and adolescents who are especially vulnerable at a particular stage of their development may discover that one of these substances reduces their inner tension and stress. A cycle of dependency on these potentially harmful substances may thus begin which, if it becomes entrenched and habituated into the developing psyche of the young person, can progress to full-on addiction.

We shall investigate the nature of each of these three sanctioned drugs to try to comprehend their unique character. This may help us to understand why the one drug suits the individual needs of a particular person.

Caffeine

At fourteen years old, Jake was a regular coffee drinker who started drinking coffee just to be cool, and because it tasted so good. He soon found it was easier to think clearly after his morning mug and he remained more alert during classes; however once the effects wore off, he felt tired and drowsy, and after school he would drink another cup to keep himself going through his afternoon activities; by evening he felt very flat and the only way he could do his homework was further coffee at night. His sleep deteriorated and a vicious cycle developed which was finally broken after nine months when he was admitted to a drug rehab centre in a state of extreme anxiety and exhaustion.

Caffeine is the most widely used consciousness-altering substance in the world. In many western countries, 80% of adults regularly drink caffeine-containing beverages, mainly in the form of coffee and tea. Younger children mainly consume caffeine in soft drinks but teens and adolescents are drinking coffee in increasing numbers.

Significant amounts of caffeine are contained in soft drinks such as Coca Cola, Pepsi and Red Bull, as well as cocoa, chocolate and medicinal preparations, sufficient to cause some symptoms of caffeine intoxication; these are heart palpitations, restlessness, agitation, anxiety and insomnia, and occur when the dose is in excess of 250mg.

The ongoing controversy over caffeinated alcoholic beverages in many countries led to the banning in the USA of a top selling drink (Four Loko, which contained alcohol, caffeine, taurine and guarana), calling caffeine an 'unsafe food additive' when added to an alcoholic beverage. The caffeine is believed to counteract the depressive effects of alcohol, keeping the individual more alert; this can lead to excess consumption of alcohol as the person tries to dull his alertness; then when the effects of caffeine wears off, the person feels the full effects of the alcohol. It is now sold without caffeine as an ingredient.[2] However, many youngsters seem to be drawn to caffeine-alcohol combinations, mixing drinks such as Red Bull with vodka or rum.

Below is a list of the average caffeine content in commonly consumed foods, drinks and drugs.[3,4] Caffeine is also found in numerous over-the-counter proprietary analgesics and migraine preparations, cold and flu remedies, diet pills and diuretics.

- Average cup of instant coffee 75–100 mg
- Average mug of instant coffee 100–150 mg
- Average cup of brewed coffee 100 mg
- Average cup of black tea 50 mg
- Green tea 30 mg
- Regular can of cola drink 30–40 mg
- Regular can of energy drink 40–80 mg
- Red Bull can 80 mg
- Plain 50 g bar of chocolate 25–50 mg
- Over-the-counter migraine preparations and caffeine stimulants 100–200 mg

Caffeine intake is naturally lower in children than in adults; in the USA children between one and nine years consume a daily average of 14–22 mg.[5] Consumption in children under eighteen years of age is about 1mg per kg, most of it coming from soft drinks and coffee.[6,7] I am not aware of representative studies that determine the average amount of caffeine or the type of caffeine consumed by children or adolescents.

What are the effects of caffeine?

We can also gain insight into caffeine's nature by observing the effects it has when consumed in different amounts:

Caffeine has no nutritional value nor is it needed physiologically. In low doses (5–100 mg), it is a central nervous stimulant causing increased alertness, a mild sense of wellbeing or euphoria and a sense of improved verbal and motor performance, enabling it to act as a positive reinforcer of behaviour. It is therefore commonly used to provide extra energy, which, for various reasons, may not be otherwise available.

However regular use of caffeine in children and adolescents may lead to a number of adverse effects: it may disrupt an already erratic sleep cycle leading to mood changes and behavioural disturbances such as aggression and impulsiveness.[8] It depletes the body's stores of calcium. Excessive consumption has been identified as a cause of headache, which usually resolves on withdrawal.[9] There are well-recognised withdrawal symptoms which include headache, insomnia, irritability, nausea, anxiety, restlessness and tremor, palpitations and raised blood pressure.[10] They are rapidly relieved by intake of caffeine, suggesting that they are genuine withdrawal symptoms. They typically start slowly, are at their worst at 1–2 days, and recede within a few days. The dependency nature of caffeine is documented in many studies.[11,12]

Caffeine enables the user to connect more effectively with his body, especially with his nervous system, allowing him to think more clearly and more cohesively.

There is a dynamic way in which the inner nature of caffeine can be experienced, in line with the methodology outlined above. First we can recall the effects caffeine has on our system, sense how this felt the last time we had a cup of coffee and recall the sensations that are now evoked in the body. We then gesture how the body feels, step aside and observe the after image we have created. This picture expresses the change in character that caffeine evokes in us. An artistic characterological representation of caffeine and other addictive agencies is included in Appendix 2, together with the methodology and the psycho-dynamic technique that underlines this approach.

Tobacco

Paolo began smoking flavoured cigarettes at the age of ten. Both his foster parents smoked and he felt very grown up taking a smoke in between computer games when they were not at home. At home they were often quarrelling which intensified Paolo's worries and anxieties. He found that smoking relaxed him and he could concentrate better on his game. In his twelfth year he started smoking cigarettes secretively, first one a day, then several times a day, frequently when his parents were fighting. He was soon craving cigarettes and would always light up before going to school, in the breaks and after school. Smoking became an habitual part of his life which he found he could not do without. This has continued into his adult years.

Tobacco has become the number one poison of pleasure for the whole of humanity. Its active ingredient, *nicotine,* is a highly toxic alkaloid that is fatal in doses of 60mg. An average cigarette contains about 9–17 mg of nicotine. In addition cigarette smoke contains carbon monoxide, a poisonous gas, and tar that is a well known carcinogen. Nicotine is a highly addictive drug just like cocaine and heroin, leading to tolerance and dependence. The World Health Organization estimates that there are 1–1.5 billion smokers worldwide; one billion of them live in developing or transitional economies, whereas the rates of smoking have declined in the developed world. Tobacco kills more than three million people annually mainly from lung disease, cancer, strokes and heart attacks. In the USA tobacco is the single most lethal carcinogen.[13]

About twenty percent of young teens aged 13–15 years smoke worldwide. In the USA approximately 29% of the population aged twelve years and older are current smokers and the rate among adolescents aged twelve to seventeen is 25%. One in two high school kids have tried smoking at some point. Tobacco is often the first drug used by young people who use alcohol and illegal drugs. Adolescents who smoke are about eight times more likely to use illicit drugs and eleven times as likely to drink heavily than non-smoking adolescents. They also tend to be more aggressive and more likely to carry weapons, suffer from mental health problems such as depression, attempt suicide and engage in high-risk sexual behaviours.

Almost all smokers start while they're young and the younger they start, the more likely they will become an adult smoker. Studies have shown that almost 90% of adults who are regular smokers started at or before the age of nineteen. This means that if people do not start using tobacco when they are young, they will most likely never start using it. And the younger they start smoking, the more likely they are to develop long-term nicotine addiction. Those most likely to begin using tobacco are young people who come from a low-income family, have fewer than two adults living in their household, who under-perform at school and have low self-image. Children are more likely to smoke if their parents and siblings smoke.[14,15] Media viewing of favourite characters enhances the risk of young people smoking.[16]

Most young people who smoke regularly are addicted to nicotine and most report that they want to quit but are unable to do so. Research shows that about three out of four high school smokers have tried to quit without success, reporting typical withdrawal symptoms; about 60% of them will still be smoking seven to nine years later.[17]

Dependence develops quickly, enhanced by social factors that encourage smoking. Children and teens are still undiscerning and impressionable and are therefore easy targets for the tobacco advertising industry. At this age they are strongly influenced by peer pressure and cannot appreciate how difficult it can be to quit; nor do they realise the damage caused by nicotine.

Cigarette smoking in children and adolescents causes serious health problems such as chronic cough with mucus production, shortness of breath, more frequent colds, flu and respiratory infections, general decline in health and nicotine addiction. In later life it leads to heart disease, strokes, cancer of the lung, chronic lung diseases such as emphysema and bronchitis, vision and hearing problems.[10]

There are other forms of tobacco favoured by teens and adolescents:

- *Smokeless tobacco* use has become a big problem especially with the increasing bans on smoking in many countries. Also known as *spit, spitless, snuff* or *chewing tobacco,* this oral form is less harmful generally but is known to cause cancers of the mouth, throat, larynx, oesophagus, stomach and pancreas, as well as gum disease, pre-cancerous lesions in the mouth (leukoplakia) and heart disease. It can also lead to nicotine addiction and users are more likely to become cigarette smokers
- *Clove cigarettes* or *kreteks* contain 60–70% tobacco and 30–40% clove extracts and other additives. They cause the same health risks as cigarettes and are more likely to induce asthma and other lung diseases.
- *Flavoured cigarettes* or *bidis,* like clove cigarettes, are used mainly as experimental cigarettes by younger smokers who believe they are safer, cleaner and more 'natural' than regular cigarettes. Because they are flavoured, colourful and hand-rolled in a tendu or temburi leaf, they are very appealing to young people. However, although they contain less tobacco than regular cigarettes, they are unfiltered and deliver more nicotine, tar, and other harmful substances such as carbon monoxide and ammonia. They are also thinner than regular cigarettes and therefore require about three times as many puffs per cigarette. This makes them at least, if not more, harmful than regular cigarettes.
- *Water pipes* or *hookahs* burn a mixture of tobacco with a variety of different flavours such as herbs, honey, molasses and dried fruit, and convey the flavoured smoke via a long hose to usually a group of smokers who engage socially as the pipe is passed around. It has been an age old tradition in Asian and Middle-Eastern countries, and has recently

become popular among younger people in Western countries. Although believed to be a safe alternative to cigarettes, the toxicity of the inhaled smoke is as high or higher than cigarette smoke because the water does not filter out many of the toxins such as carbon monoxide, nicotine, tar and heavy metals.

- *Small cigars* look similar to cigarettes, are sold in packs, are often flavoured and are cheaper than cigarettes because they are classed as cigars and not taxed or regulated like cigarettes. This makes them more accessible to younger kids, leading in recent years to an equal or greater use than cigarettes. They are as addictive and harmful as cigarettes.

What are the effects of nicotine?

Tobacco appears to improve attention, learning, reaction time and problem solving through its stimulating effects on the nervous system. However it also appears to have a sedating affect on certain areas in the central nervous system. It is reported to lift moods, decrease tension and reduce depressive feelings.[10] Tobacco has a powerful stimulating effect on the blood circulation and the heart but not on the respiration. This leads to a mild lack of oxygen (hypoxia) in the blood which causes a subliminal shortness of breath and a faint but constant state of anxiety; this again causes the heart to speed up, leading to further hypoxia and anxiety. Nicotine also relaxes the tension in the muscular system, giving the illusion to the smoker that by smoking his subliminal breathlessness and low grade anxiety will abate. This relaxes the muscular system but not the cardio-respiratory system, leading to a repetitive cycle and physiological dependency on top of the psychological one is created. The reduction in nicotine in the body leads to a mild withdrawal effect that is alleviated each time a cigarette is smoked.

Physiologically, the inhaled nicotine triggers chemical reactions in nerve endings in the central nervous system and skeletal muscles, leading to increased heart rate, alertness and faster reaction times. Dopamine, a neurohormone associated with pleasure, is also released, which may reinforce the smoking habit.[18] Nicotine and cocaine activate similar patterns of neurons, which supports the idea that common neural substrates exist for the addictive properties of nicotine and other drugs.[19]

The priming of these neuro receptors by nicotine may pave the way for the subsequent use of other addiction-forming drugs.[20]

Children growing up in an electronic age are exposed to a continuous over-stimulation of their senses and a constant overload of their nervous system. An intellectual and academic education further burdens their neuro-sensory system. They experience this subconsciously as a disquieting pressure and will seek ways of alleviating this internal stress. They may search for a chemical substance that alleviates the pressure on their nervous systems and discover that tobacco does just that. Tobacco is able to do this because it strongly stimulates the cardio-vascular system and re-equilibrates the nervous system thereby creating for a brief period some measure of equilibrium.[21] Unfortunately, once again, an addictive and toxic agent is used as a substitute to fulfil real needs (pressure on the nervous system) which should be addressed in other more healthy ways.

We can connect with tobacco experientially when we recall the effects tobacco has on our system (if we have ever smoked); we sense how this felt the last time we smoked a cigarette and remember the sensations that were evoked in the body. Once again, we gesture how the body feels, then step aside and observe the picture of our body (see Appendix 2).

Alcohol

Peter was a highly sensitive child who masked his vulnerability with an abrasive and aggressive outer façade. It was a common thing for him to have a sip of his parents' drinks who were both regular drinkers. He had his first alcoholic drink at the age of ten and by age twelve would secretly raid the family liquor cabinet when he felt upset or tense. Because alcohol was so freely available at home, he would have a few drinks before a party or disco. He would often have a drink after school and by fifteen years he was binge drinking at parties. He was part of a group of assertive kids who smoked and drank alcohol. His health and performance at school started to deteriorate. On one occasion he was taken, comatose, to hospital with alcohol intoxication. Things finally came to a head when he crashed his parents' car, inebriated without a driver's licence. Law enforcement compelled him to undergo psychotherapeutic counselling and to enter an alcohol rehab programme.

Alcohol is, after tobacco, the second most widely used addictive substance in the world. The World Health Organization estimates that there are about two billion people worldwide who consume alcoholic beverages and 76.3 million with diagnosable alcohol-use disorders.[22] In the USA over 50% of all adults are current users of alcohol. In Europe alone, alcohol consumption was responsible for over fifty-five thousand deaths among young people aged 15–29 years. In the USA, forty thousand people die annually from alcohol abuse (compared to four thousand from heroin).[23] Alcohol consumption is the leading risk factor for disease in low-mortality developing countries, and the third largest risk factor in developed countries, in 1999. In South Africa it is the third largest contributor to death and disability after unsafe sexually transmitted infections and interpersonal violence.[24]

Alcohol is a major factor in the three leading causes of death in youth: suicide, motor vehicle accidents and homicide. It is also linked to two-thirds of all sexual assaults and date rapes of teens and college students.[25]

It is the drug of choice among youth in developed countries and therefore a leading public health problem. Approximately 40% of children between twelve to fourteen years of age use alcohol occasionally. The average age of a child's first drink appears to be lower than ever before: in 1965 it was 17.5 years, in 2003 it was fourteen years, today it is twelve years. From sixteen years, the consumption pattern is similar to that of an adult. Research has shown that youth who begin drinking before age fifteen are four times more likely to develop alcohol dependence at some time in their lives compared with those who have their first drink at age twenty or older.[26]

Although alcohol abuse and dependency are more likely to be preceded by early experimentation, social drinking and misuse, it is still not clear whether starting to drink at an early age actually causes alcoholism.

What is incontestable is the fact that alcohol is a toxic substance that can cause damage to various systems if consumption has been prolonged or heavy. The ethanol content of various drinks varies considerably ranging from 2.5% (weak beer) to 55% (strong spirits). The average alcohol content in a standard beer is 5%, in wine is 12% and in liquor is 40%.

A proportion of youth drink intensively, often consuming four to five drinks or more at one time. This pattern of heavy drinking, known as binge drinking, corresponds to raising the blood alcohol concentration

(BAC) to 0.08 grams percent or above in about two hours. The normal BAC is 0.01–0.02 grams percent. This equates on average to five or more standard alcoholic drinks on the same occasion. Nearly 20 percent of twelve to twenty-year-olds are considered binge drinkers. In the USA, this amounts to nearly 1 million high school students.[27] Furthermore, frequent binge drinkers are more likely to use other drugs such as marijuana and cocaine, engage in risky sex encounters and perform poorly in school.[28]

What are the effects of alcohol consumption?

Common experience – physiological effects

Many of us will recall the first effects of a few beers or glasses of wine as a pleasant and comfortable feeling of freedom with loss of inhibitions, release of emotions and a greater sense of power. The stimulated heart, blood circulation and respiration allows everything to flow – speech, warmth and emotions. Our higher human functions of rational, critical thinking and fine discriminatory sensing diminish.

As the intoxification increases, metabolic functions activated by the enhanced blood flow overwhelm neuro-sensory functions leading to depression of these capacities as well as nausea and vomiting. The human being regresses to a more child like state, progressively losing the power of speech (slurring), walking (loss of coordination), standing (loss of balance, dizziness), vision (double vision) and thinking, eventually falling into sleep and oblivion.

Alcohol is absorbed rapidly into the blood stream, significant amounts being absorbed from the stomach lining especially if the stomach is empty. The effects will last for several hours depending on how much and how quickly it was ingested, as well as the quantity and nature of food taken with it. Because female bodies contain less water, they will absorb alcohol faster and produce a higher concentration in the blood. This will lead to the effects manifesting more rapidly and lasting longer.

Health risks

The brain continues to develop during adolescence, with refinement of pathways and circuits, especially in the frontal lobe, until age 16. Extensive research over twenty years by the American Medical Association showed that excessive alcohol during this developmental period can result in long-term and irreversible brain damage. Short-term or moderate drinking leads to neuro-psychological deficits and impairs cognitive function by damaging two key areas of the brain: the hippocampus, which handles many types of memory and learning, is affected most in teen drinkers, while the pre-frontal area, which play an important role in forming adult personality and behaviour, is most affected during adolescence. Deficits in vocabulary and general information, memory and sleep disturbances as well as an impaired ability to delay gratification, regulate emotions and appreciate future consequences of actions were found; there was also an increased risk of social problems, depression, suicidal thoughts and violence.[10,29]

However, young drinkers are able to consume much larger quantities of alcohol than adults before experiencing negative effects. This is believed to be due to the differences between the adult brain and the brain of the maturing adolescent and may explain the high rates of binge drinking among young adults.

Liver damage, indicated by elevated liver enzymes, has been found in some adolescents who consume alcohol.[30] Those who were overweight or obese showed raised liver enzymes with only moderate drinking.[31]

Puberty, a time of rapid growth, is associated with hormonal changes that lead to increased production of sex hormones, cortisol and growth factors that are critical for the healthy development of organ systems. Alcohol consumption during this period may upset this delicate hormonal balance, leading to disturbances in normal development of the musculo-skeletal system and other organs.[32] Studies in animals also show that consuming alcohol during puberty adversely affects the maturation of the reproductive system.

Binge drinking can be highly dangerous or even lethal. In the USA, drinking-related accidental deaths among college students have been creeping upward – from 1,440 in 1998 to 1,825 in 2005.[33] In the UK, death rates due to acute intoxication have doubled in the last twenty years.[34]

Psycho-social effects

Drinking and driving is a major cause of motor vehicle accidents that are the leading cause of death in the age group between fifteen to twenty years. Fatal crashes involving drivers who consume alcohol are twice as common in sixteen to twenty-year-olds compared to drivers of twenty-one years and older.[35,36]

Depression and stress are aggravated by alcohol consumption and *suicide,* or its attempt, is a common occurrence in heavy drinkers. Suicide is the third leading cause of death among people between the ages of fourteen and twenty-five. In one study, 37 percent of fifteen-year-old girls who drank heavily reported attempting suicide, compared with 11 percent who did not drink.[37]

Sexual assault, including rape, frequently involves the use of alcohol by the offender, the victim or both, and increases the risk of sexual assault.

Sexual offences occur most commonly against women in late adolescence and early adulthood, and frequently within the context of a date. In one study, approximately 10 percent of female high school students reported having been raped.[38]

High-risk sex, through multiple partners or unprotected sex, has been associated with adolescent alcohol use. This is also an age group where the consequences of high-risk sex, such as teenage pregnancy, sexually transmitted diseases, and HIV/AIDS are common. According to a recent study, the link between high-risk sex and drinking is affected by the quantity of alcohol consumed.[39]

Violence: there is a well established association between alcohol and violence. Although alcohol consumption does not always lead to violent behaviour, a review of recent research has shown that 62% of violent offenders were intoxicated at the time of their offence.[40,41]

We can enter empathically into the functional nature of alcohol by sensing the effects it has on us. We give expression to this awareness by acting out the experience, then observing our actions and catching the picture of alcohol in us like a photo image (see Appendix 2).

Why do some children drink?

There are many factors that will determine why some teens and adolescents drink alcohol, and why others don't:

Children and youth who have a sensitive and vulnerable disposition seem more likely to drink alcohol and do so often at a very early age (before twelve years of age). They may mask their sensitivity through disruptive or aggressive antisocial behaviour or manifest it through withdrawal, anxiety and depression. Alcohol use in young people is also often associated with impulsive, defiant and other types of anti-social behaviour.

Pre-puberty and the threshold of puberty open the child to new challenges and with it also new dangers. With the awakening of his soul life at puberty as described in Chapter 2, the teenager begins to experience a new sense of power surging through both his body and mind, a power that wishes to express itself in a host of new experiences which announce his new found independence. This brings with it a need to break out of his protected home environment and to seek to explore activities that will allow him to discover more of who he really is. At the same time, the forces of his soul life – his desires, sensuality, sexuality, emotionality and intellectuality – take on a life of their own, creating new needs that drive him to seek their gratification. In accordance with his nature and what he meets in his environment, he will therefore open himself to new experiences and try out new things. For some teens, thrill-seeking means taking risks which might include experimenting with alcohol. Because his power of judgment and discernment are still unformed and because this is a time when the protection of parental authority is often rejected, the young adolescent is more vulnerable to succumbing to a host of temptations. And alcohol seems to be the one that is most appropriate for this time.

One may well ask why alcohol is one of the first drugs to be used by young people, beginning frequently around puberty. We may find a clue to this question when we look at the use of alcohol in antiquity.

It is well known that wine was used in the cult of Dionysus during the Greek civilisation from approximately 700 BC. Large quantities of wine were consumed in ritualistic and orgiastic cults of celebration, where animals were sacrificed in communal rites. The participants in these rituals were instructed to exercise self-control over the large amounts of alcohol consumed, in this way gaining mastery over their 'inner animals'. Rudolf Steiner describes how the cult of Dionysus evolved from the wisdom of the Greek mystery centres.[42] This cult had the mission of cutting the human being off from his time-honoured connection to his spiritual home and drawing him down into the material world, whereby his soul life became more immersed in his body. It thus helped to prepare humanity for the evolutionary transformation into self-individuation and to develop capacities to control the animal nature that emerged through the deeper fusion with the body.[43]

Puberty is the time when the child loses his heavenly connection and falls into earthly matter: limbs get heavier, the voice drops, the body becomes ungainly and clumsy. It is also the time when the psychological forces of desire and feeling awaken, and manifest themselves powerfully through the whole body. In the years that follow, the adolescent needs to explore these awakened soul forces in order that he may gradually learn to control their animalistic power.

Is it possible that many adolescents are challenged by alcohol to get to know the raw unrestrained power of the soul and, like Dionysus in the Greek era, to wrestle with these forces in the striving to control them? Children in this vulnerable time, however, do not have the individuated strength of self to resist the heightened forces induced by alcohol, and can easily be overcome by this false sense of power. Because they are unable to work on the untamed forces of the soul through their own strength, and because the will to harness the lower needs of the soul have not been exercised through the healthy developmental process, a life-long disposition for dependency can be created

Before puberty, when the soul life is not fully awakened, alcohol is especially dangerous, since it awakens the soul forces prematurely leading to a kind of premature birth. The effect on the child is similar to what could happen when a firearm is put into his hands. These forces unleashed before puberty are very difficult to control in later life resulting in an overall weakening of self-control.

Environmental influences

The environment in which a sensitive and vulnerable child grows up will undoubtedly influence whether he chooses to drink alcohol. The influence of parents and peers play a role in alcohol use. For example, children who grow up with parents who drink frequently and who view drinking favourably, will tend to start drinking early and drink larger quantities.[44] Adolescent girls who socialise with older men are more likely to use alcohol and other drugs.[45] Adolescents who mix with peers who drink will be at greater risk of drinking alcohol.

The attitudes and expectations of teens have been shown to influence drinking behaviour; for instance a teenager who expects drinking to be a cool experience is more likely to drink than one who does not.[46] Attitudes and beliefs about alcohol appear to be formed early in life. Children younger than nine generally regard drinking alcohol in a negative light, but by about age thirteen, their belief system shifts and they view alcohol more positively. Adolescents who drink excessively place great value on the positive merits of alcohol.

Positive beliefs and attitudes towards alcohol are aggressively promoted through the media; research has found that teens and adolescents who are attracted by adverts for alcohol are more positive towards drinking and want to purchase products with these attractive logos.[47] It is not clear whether media promotion leads to under-age drinking.

Genetics and brain factors

There is some evidence that hereditary or genetic factors are also involved. Children of alcoholic family members are between four and ten times more likely to become alcoholics than children who have no such relationships; they are also more likely to start drinking early and to develop alcohol problems more quickly. Current research is attempting to identify the actual genes involved in alcohol dependency and has found specific regions on chromosomes that correlate with a risk for alcoholism.[48]

Research has shown that children of alcoholic parents may have subtle brain differences, both in structure and function, which could be indicators for developing alcohol problems later in life. These neurological differences have also featured prominently in people with behavioural traits such as antisocial personality disorder, and conduct or impulsivity disorders, that also manifest in alcoholics.[49] There thus seems to be some correlation between neurological structure and function, and personality and behaviour patterns, manifesting in particular in later alcohol use.[50]

The big question asked by natural scientists however is: what comes first? Does the genetic and neurological make-up of a person lead to an anxious and vulnerable disposition that, around puberty, results in using alcohol to alleviate anxiety; or does the psychological disposition at an early age determine the neurological and genetic make-up?

From an holistic perspective the genome certainly appears to determine physical and chemical characteristics such as skin colour, body size and physiological function, but psycho-spiritual attributes such as personality type and intellectual capacity have never been proven to arise from the physical constitution. It is only a materialistic view of the human being that would give this any consideration. When the soul and spirit are accorded their own independent reality and existence, interconnected with the body as a dynamic and functional whole, the significance of the genome becomes limited to the bio-chemical and physiological realm of the human being.

It is probable that drinking behaviour reflects a complex interplay between a number of factors – inherited, dispositional, developmental and environmental.

Understanding the nature of sanctioned drugs

Body-soul-spirit-continuum

We have described the human being as an interactive continuum of body, soul and spirit, where the psyche or soul is the mediating link between body and spirit. These three realms are by no means separate and distinct from one another, constantly interacting psychosomatically and psycho-spiritually: thus the physical relaxing effects that alcohol has on the body will also cause the psychological feelings of pleasure and comfort, while soul passion and enthusiasm will fire a person to attain the highest spiritual ideals.

We saw that the *body* belongs to the world of matter, and as an object of matter can be perceived by the organs of sense such as sight and hearing. It provides the physical foundation for the soul to function in the physical material world, while the soul lifts physical existence into the realm of experience. The *soul* as the domain of inner experience serves as a vessel in which the spirit can work, that in turn brings the gifts of the spiritual world down into the realm of soul experience. The *spirit* belongs to a higher reality where the universal law of the good and the true prevail. Into all three realms, the *Self* or *I* works and exists as an individuating, integrating and unifying force (see Figure 3).[51]

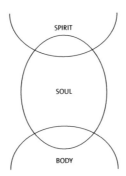

Figure 3. Body-soul-spirit continuum in the human being.

It is common experience that all drugs have an effect on the human constitution, affecting all three aspects in quite specific ways. The effects of caffeine, tobacco and alcohol can be summarised as:

- caffeine is a central nervous stimulant causing increased alertness and improved intellectual performance;
- tobacco has a stimulating action on the blood circulation and the heart, and a mild euphoric effect;
- alcohol enhances blood flow and intensifies metabolic functions; neuro-sensory functions and cognitive capacities are depressed but emotions are enhanced.

All three socially accepted drugs, fully sanctioned by our world civilisation, *draw the soul more deeply down into the body,* caffeine more into the head region, tobacco more into the rhythmic heart-circulatory region and alcohol more into the metabolic-blood region.[52]

Three primary systems

Viewed dynamically, there are three primary systems that encompass the whole biological nature of the human being and provide the physical foundation for all psychological functions. It is a view that allows for an integrated understanding of the human constitution as a being of body, soul and spirit.

The *neuro-sensory system* is the information-receiving centre, enabling the soul functions of *thinking* and *sensing* to operate in the physical material world. To sense the world, sense organs and nerve organs are required; to think and reflect, the healthy functioning brain is needed. The primary function of the neuro-sensory system is to bring to awareness and mirror for us the sense-perceptible world. It is the cool, calm and passive side of our system that contracts the world into our internal centre.

The *metabolic motor system* generates metabolism, movement and the energy needed for the will-based functions of the psyche to become active. Through all metabolic activities, which include the blood, digestive, liver, hormonal and loco-motor system, we become active and mobile in the world and in our inner life. It is the warm, mobile and active pole of our system that opens us up and extends us out into the world.

The *rhythmic system* comprises the integrated totality of all rhythmic activities in the human organism. The cardiovascular-respiratory systems constitute the primary rhythmic organs of the body which alternate the polar activities of contraction and expansion, systole and diastole, inspiration and expiration, bringing the human organism into harmonious equilibrium. The rhythmic system is that system that harmonises the two diametrically opposed systems mentioned above, bringing the centripetally orientated neuro-sensory system into harmony with the centrifugally orientated metabolic motor system. The rhythmic nature of this system is finely tuned to our life of feeling – feelings affect our breathing and vice versa – and provides the dynamic foundation for the fourth soul function of *feeling*.[40]

CAFFEINE	–	NEURO-SENSORY SYSTEM
TOBACCO	–	RHYTHMIC SYSTEM
ALCOHOL	–	METABOLIC MOTOR SYSTEM

Two polar disease tendencies

There are fundamentally two essential disease tendencies or dispositions that are at the root of all disease processes in the human being and in the world. One is the tendency for the material element to become too dominant, the other is for the spiritual element to become too powerful.

The *material disposition draws us more into our bodies, into our earthly material nature,* giving us the experience of a power that draws on living matter, cold reason and intellect. It is the cynical egoistic scientist in us who craves measurable earthly realities and regards the world mechanistically, devoid of soul and spirit. It lives in the firm, solid, secure structures of the earth. It is the power that rules our Western material- and capitalist-driven culture.

The *spiritual tendency draws us away from our physical bodies and from the earth,* making us too spiritual and driving us to ever greater heights of creative power, knowledge and beauty; it is the artist, the creative, desiring, impulsive and wilful nature in us. It lives in the air, the light and the warmth and it shuns the earth. Eastern spirituality and culture tends to be driven by this power.

A preponderance of matter expresses itself anatomically in hard and firm body tissues (skeleton), pathologically in all the cold hardening sclerotic diseases (atherosclerosis, clotting tendencies, arthritis), in the heaviness of fear and doubt based depressive illnesses and the constrictive nature of obsessive compulsive and neurotic conditions, in all centripetal tendencies that draw the human being too strongly towards his physical centre. This is the dynamic of the neuro-sensory system working without restriction.

Predominance of spirit manifests anatomically in softer, mobile fluid, airy and warm tissues (glandular, blood), pathologically in the warm dissolving inflammatory conditions (febrile illnesses, inflammations of all kinds, TB, pneumonia), in the expansive nature of illusory and hallucinatory illnesses (mania, psychoses), in all centrifugal tendencies that drive the human being away from his physical centre towards the spirit. Here we find the dynamic of the metabolic blood and motor system active without limitation.

Pneumo-psychosomatic dynamics

All three sanctioned drugs draw the soul more deeply down into the body and because each one appears to work in a different psychosomatic realm, the particular effects of each drug will be different. We may therefore postulate that:

- *caffeine* drives the soul forces more strongly into the neuro-sensory system, empowering the cognitive life to become more active;
- *tobacco* leads the soul life preferentially into the rhythmic system, thereby impacting more strongly into the feeling and emotive activities of the psyche;
- *alcohol* pushes the soul forces down into the blood and thence into the metabolic and motor systems, driving the *Self* progressively out of the body. This leaves a lower soul life in command of a bodily nature empowered by the blood forces. No longer controlled by the *Self*, the soul is free to experience without inhibitions, pleasure and displeasure, drives, passions and desires.

Understanding the sanctioned drug-dependent youth

Working again with the methodological approach outlined in Chapter 2, we put aside our personal issues and prejudices towards these substances, open up to the young person in our focus with interest and respect, and endeavour to understand the child in the keen manner described before. We are also attentive to the developmental road map that will orientate us to the specific nature and needs of this child in this phase of his life.

In this way we discover that Jake, Paolo and Peter all found a socially accepted drug that helped them deal with their inner discomfort. Their real needs were not addressed: Jake used caffeine because he needed to be a cool guy and liked to impress, then he used it to take away his tiredness; Paolo became addicted to cigarettes because he needed to relax and found that smoking removed his anxiety and tenseness; Peter drank to cover up his insecurities and lack of confidence, because he needed desperately to appear strong and in control. When we look more deeply into the biographies of each child, we discover essentially the same dynamic: that unresolved inner needs lead to psycho-emotional discomfort which induces a search for something that alleviates the pain. Caffeine, nicotine and ethanol become for these youngsters the repetitive, short-term addictive substitute that is able to ease the inner discomfort for a brief period (see box).

Unfulfilled primary need ➤ pain ➤ blocking of the need ➤ ensuing discomfort ➤ the finding and adopting of a substitute gratification ➤ appeases the pain briefly ➤ secondary need ➤ dependency on substitute agency

---

Based on the fact that each of these three drugs affects a different constitutional region, we may well ask whether there is a rational explanation why the child selects specifically one or other drug to alleviate his inner pain. We shall take up this question in the next chapter when we examine the various illicit drug substances and the specific effects that they have on the child's constitution.

Helping youngsters with sanctioned substance addictions

The first step to helping children deal effectively with dependency on these substances is to gain a clear understanding of the nature of addiction and the inner dynamics as to why this particular child uses this particular substance to gratify his needs. To do this properly, as stated repeatedly above, one has to remove one's own personal blocks and dispositions regarding these issues. Check the feelings of discomfort you may be carrying towards the child's dependency and decide where they belong. What is your attitude to these sanctioned drugs? Children are strongly influenced by parental attitudes and behaviour and will often copy or rebel against them.

One will then need to determine the phase of development of the child, the kind of child you are dealing with and the nature of the child's environment.

Special attention should be given to the needs and feelings of ongoing discomfort, dissatisfaction, deprivation, frustration and distress in the inner life of the child or adolescent, especially from pubescence onwards. Leaving these feelings unattended will often provoke the child's neediness to search for ways to block the pain.

The earliest signs of interest for these drugs should be closely monitored, the degree of dependency should be carefully assessed and any addictive tendencies need to be attended to as soon as possible in the most sensitive and respectful way possible. One should also be aware of changes in health or behaviour patterns. If such early signs had been detected in the cases of Jake, Paolo and Peter, much could have been done to prevent their full-blown addictions.

Next, one seeks to acquire an experiential profile of the child by the method described in Chapter 2. By entering into the inner nature of the child through one's own experience, one will gain insight into the help and support needed.

Each level of dependency will require appropriate management. In all situations, effective communication based on trust, respect and interest is crucial to creating a partnership that will bring about the self-reflection needed for change to happen. The conditions and ethical guidelines described in Chapter 3 will actively support this process.

In cases of addiction to one of the three sanctioned substances, an individual therapeutic programme will need to be constructed. Building on the partnership created and supported by family, school and community, the client needs to be encouraged to find the motivation, commitment and accountability that will free him from dependency. Clearly negotiated contracts and short-term time frames create the structures necessary to steer the client through the difficult phase of withdrawal.

The therapeutic programme may include dietary planning, intravenous nutritional and detox interventions, oral medication with natural substances and optional therapies such as massage, art therapy, dance and movement therapy.

Counselling is an essential part of the therapeutic programme.

Peter came to his first counselling session feeling deeply remorseful for the damage caused by his car accident, to the other driver of the car, his parents and to his own life. He was keen to change his ways and it was therefore easy to establish a gwood partnership with him and to create together a way forward. It was more difficult engaging with his parents, who denied they had an alcohol problem or that the free availability of alcohol in the home and their behaviour around alcohol were important contributing factors. A separate session was needed for them to engage with the process and become part of the therapeutic team. They agreed to curtail their drinking habits and to remove the exposure of liquor in the home.

A therapeutic contract was negotiated with Peter, drawn up and signed. He agreed to change his diet and take oral medicines to support his liver which had been weakened by alcohol abuse. He undertook to steadily reduce his smoking over a six week period and to unconditionally stop drinking any form of alcohol. He committed himself to weekly sessions of psychophonetic counselling for the next six weeks.

Peter soon realised he was also addicted to smoking, and needed alcohol to give him those feelings of self-importance and empowerment. He could see that deep inside him there was an insecure and vulnerable person who lacked the confidence needed to maintain his position among his peer group. Acknowledging this part of himself was the step needed to embrace and care for himself. This required him to find someone within who was genuinely strong and compassionate enough to care for himself. Finding this resource was the key he needed to overcoming the addictive need for nicotine or ethanol. He came to see these substances as false agencies that seduced him into needing to be gratified by them and recognised the enormous damage that these substances had already caused him and others.

Caffeine, nicotine and ethanol come in the guise of socially acceptable and pleasure creating substances that disguise their potential danger as addictive substances. They have become popular friends of society that have ingratiated themselves into our lives, concealing their true identity as potentially dangerous playmates. Adults who are in command of their own choices can exercise control and restraint over these pleasurable acquaintances, keeping them in their proper place and preventing them from over-exceeding their seductive nature. Children and youth, however, do not yet have the maturity to resist the power these substances bestow on them, placing them at the mercy of their addictive nature.

Chapter 6. Illicit Substance Abuse

I have seen the terrible destruction that drugs wreak on the lives of children and their loved ones. I have felt the enormous power that these substances have on the human soul. I have experienced the strength needed to overcome this alien power. Needy children and youth who are exposed to these false prophets and parasites of our time do not have the insight or strength to resist these seductive forces. I wish to explore ways of understanding these drugs. I wish to find the means of helping vulnerable children free themselves from drug entrapment and drug slavery.

—

South Africa has become a major drug haven for world drug markets. As a result, children and youth are increasingly exposed to old and new types of drugs. They are freely available on many street corners, in schools and malls, at parties, nightclubs, raves and in drug houses. Current South African statistics indicate that two schools in every five report the presence of drug merchants on the premises during school hours. Drug contacts can be found readily and needy teenagers and adolescents are easy prey. Such drug conduits are present in every country, to a greater or lesser extent. These drugs become dangerous and illusory gratifications for vulnerable young people, wreaking havoc in their lives and those of their families.

This chapter will examine the spectrum of illicit drugs and will explore the particular way each drug provides a specific and appropriate gratification for the individual needs of the drug user.

Experiencing drug abuse and drug addiction

What is your experience of the use and abuse of illicit drugs? For most of us, our experience of drug abuse and addiction comes from the outside, what we have heard about, what we have read, or in some cases what we have seen by observing others using the drugs. Some of us know about drug misuse through direct contact with a drug dependent person. And there are some who know about it from the inside, those who are trapped or have been trapped in the dangerous cycle of drug dependency.

Whatever the context of our experience with drugs, any exposure is imprinted on our psyche and this now becomes our first hand experience.

What is your experience of addiction? Drugs are usually the first association when one thinks of addiction. Is this because the drug is a tangible entity, with a specific profile that may be glorified or demonised, and produces a known and predictable gratification that can lead to vicious dependency? Addiction to other agents or activities is perhaps not so concrete and visible.

Our human experience constitutes that inner realm we have called *psyche* or *soul*. This is our starting point for acquiring any kind of knowledge and in this chapter for gaining insight into the addictions caused by illicit substances. We also need to recall that it is the psyche where addictions play out their life drama. We return again to the body-soul-spirit continuum as the reality of the human constitution.

The human constitution

In the previous chapter we described the human being as an interactive continuum of body, soul and spirit. This has to be visualised as a dynamic and continuous interplay of forces where activities of one sphere interact with those of the other two. For instance, the desire for food and its enjoyment (a psychological process) takes place concurrently with the digestion of this food (a physiological process). At the same time, our higher intentions and moral conscience – a higher spiritual activity – will dictate what kind of food will best keep us healthy.

We may regard the principal states of consciousness – waking, dreaming and sleeping – as an outcome of this interweaving continuum of body, soul and spirit.

In the waking state there is an active engagement of psycho-spiritual activities with bodily processes; we utilise our thinking, feeling and perceptive capacities to interact with the world and our bodies; we become conscious and wake up to the outer world. *Psyche* connects with *body*. When these psychological activities cease, we lose consciousness and fall either into the deep sleep or the dreaming state where we are no longer aware of our bodies or the outer world. We fall asleep to the outer world and our bodies. *Psyche* withdraws from the *body* (see Figure 4).

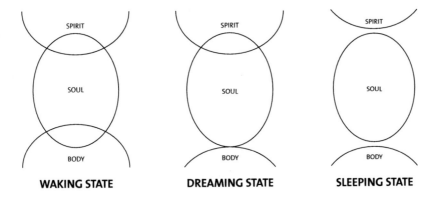

Figure 4. States of human consciousness.

While we dream we are dimly aware of an imaginative realm where anything is possible; after we awaken, we may reflect on the dream and know that it is a state of consciousness that is clearly distinct from the waking and the deep sleeping state.

The interconnection of body, soul and spirit may thus be said to determine these three distinct levels of consciousness. In other words, the activities and movements of the one sphere in relation to the other will determine to a great degree these different states of consciousness.[1]

Earthly experience-cosmic experience

We experience life in two main ways: either through the agency of our body or through our psycho-spiritual organisation. We see or smell some delicious food, taste it and sense the pleasure it gives the body; at the same time or afterwards we may reflect on the meal, fantasise about it, feel emotionally satisfied by it or recall another such meal.

The first may be called *earthly experience* where we engage our earthly material nature, that is, our sense organs, with the outer physical world, which also includes our physical body, and then engage our bodily nature by eating and digesting the meal. The second I call *cosmic experience*

101

where we are active inwardly in an immaterial world of thinking, feeling, memory and imagination. Earthly experience meets an outer world of form and structure that can be measured, weighed and numbered according to the laws of the physical world. Cosmic experience lives in an inner world of formless mobility, fantasy and creativity governed by laws that belong to an immaterial cosmic world.

On the basis of such experience we discover that there exist two contrasting paradigms of experience that allow us to view the world and ourselves from an outer earthly or inner cosmic point of view.

Our physical nature belongs to the earthly world; our soul-spiritual nature belongs to the cosmic world. Our physical nature embraces the composite world of matter: all things solid, fluid, gaseous and even warmth that can be sensed by fine sensory organs of the body. We are also connected to the world of matter through activities and functions that bring about mineralisation, densification, contraction, cooling down, material concentration and centripetal action. These are forces that belong to the earthly world. On the other hand our soul-spiritual nature connects us to super-sensible dimensions that can be experienced by higher sensory functions, feelings, thoughts and impulses of the will. Those bodily activities that disconnect us from the material world, such as de-mineralisation, dissolution of substances, expansion and centrifugal activities which disperses matter, as well as soul-spiritual activities that engage with the immaterial imaginative world, are part of the cosmic world.

Children and adolescents may be characterised very broadly according to these two categories: the one type may be called the *earthly child*, the other type the *cosmic child*.[2]

The earthly child is usually a pale, small-headed child with a firm dry body and long limbs, who has lost her childhood softness. She cannot concentrate well, is restless and lacks creative fantasy. She is good at arithmetic and reading but hopeless in the arts and composition. She lives strongly in her body.

The cosmic child has a large or domed head with a child-like roundish face, soft warm body and weak short legs. She generally has a warm pleasant disposition, an active imagination, leading to dreaming and fanciful ideas; she experiences the world more in pictures and is therefore a good artist but weak in analytical activities (arithmetic, grammar). These children live strongly in their soul and spirit.

Similarly, there are two principal disease tendencies or dispositions that result in functional, psychological and structural disease processes in the human being. We became acquainted with them in the previous chapter. One is a preponderance of the material element, the other a predominance of the soul-spiritual element.

We saw that the *material disposition draws us down into earthly experience*, connecting us more with our physical nature, our cold reason and hardened intellect; it may convey an experience of power that draws on the physical world of matter. The nature of earth is formed, compact, and constrictive. Soul and spirit become overwhelmed by the earthly, becoming harder, heavier, cooler, denser and more earthbound. It is as if soul and spirit are drawn down into the body.

The *spiritual disposition draws us away from earthly experience* and our own physical bodies, into an immaterial realm of light and warmth, of beauty, imagination and creativity. The nature of cosmic is unformed, immaterial and expansive. Soul and spirit, unencumbered by the body, withdraw from the body (see Figure 5).

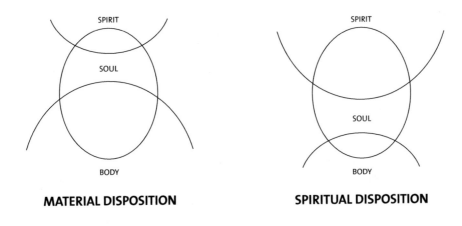

MATERIAL DISPOSITION   SPIRITUAL DISPOSITION

Figure 5. Dispositions of the human being.

As we saw before, the medical sciences, such as anatomy, physiology, pathology and therapeutics, can all be classified according to these two extremes. Tissues such as bone and cartilage are more earthly than blood and lymph; systole – the contraction phase of the heart – is an earthly functionality compared to the relaxing diastolic phase which is more cosmic; illnesses that harden the body such as arthritis are earthly pathologies compared to inflammation which softens and liquifies matter.[3]

An approach to understanding the illicit drugs

Earthly drugs, cosmic drugs

Illicit drugs may also be viewed according to these two categories, allowing deep insight into their nature. In the previous chapter we described how all drugs affect the human constitution, bringing about distinct changes in the body-soul-spirit continuum. Certain drugs draw the individual's soul nature more into her body; these may be called the *earthly drugs*. Such drugs may be used more by an earthly child because they feel at home with these earthly effects. Other drugs lift the soul out of the body; we may call these the *cosmic drugs*. They may be used by a cosmic child because it corresponds to her current needs. On the other hand, a cosmic child may feel instinctively that an earthly substance like coffee balances out her nature and brings her down to earth, just as an earthly child may find that a cosmic substance like sugar lifts her out of her heaviness.

We may explore the nature of these drugs using the same approach that we have used in previous chapters to understand the nature of a particular child.

With unreserved openness, curiosity and interest for these substances, we direct our observation to the particular substance and learn as much as possible about its physical, chemical, historical and pharmacological profile; this information can be obtained from any authoritative reference source. We can also explore the effects the drug has on the user. How does her character change when she takes this substance? At the same time we notice the effect it has on our feelings and sensations as well as the meaning we attach to all the phenomena we observe. We are looking for an essential common profile for all the many phenomena that we can observe.

If we are in a position to observe a person under the influence of the drug or if we are in the company of someone who has used the drug and can share her experience with us, we can go even further. We can use the power of *imitation* to penetrate more deeply into the nature of the drug itself as it affects the user. How does it entice the user before it enters her system? What does it do to the user when it is in her system? Who or what does she become when the drug is inside of her? We mimic what we observe in this person, try and sense what she experiences and then find a gesture which accurately portrays or imitates the inner experience. We then step aside and observe imaginatively this picture we have created. But something very specific has created this form. Just as a tissue which is crumpled must have the hand which crumples it, so the drug user who is emboldened by the use of speed (amphetamine), must have the 'hand' of speed that has created this new personality structure. We can visualise the way speed transforms the personality and we can then physically enter its nature and dramatically express its activity as we imaginatively experience it. Thus the amphetamine is revealed to me as an extremely wilful, energising and physically empowering personality; cocaine works in a similar manner with powerful enhancement of the cognitive faculties; marijuana is a softer, more relaxed and fine feeling being; while heroin is an other-worldly power that can evoke the most ecstatic and euphoric feelings and sensations.

In this way we can gain deep and intimate experience of all the illicit drugs. An artistic representation of some of the illicit drugs is included in Appendix 2, together with more details regarding the underlying methodology and the psycho-developmental technique utilised. It must be stated quite clearly that this is a methodology that, like any other, can only be properly applied with the requisite training and practice.[4]

A living experience of these drugs in the way described above, as well as an investigation of their nature and actions, justify this classification into earthly and cosmic drugs.

Earthly drugs

Jody grew up in a working class home where her parents were mostly out working. She was the youngest of six children , a shy, sensitive girl whose parents had little time to attend to her emotional needs. Her other siblings were busy with their lives and had no time for her and as a child with little self-confidence, she struggled to cope with the challenges of growing up. When she was nine years old, her father had an affair and left home. Her mother struggled desperately to hold the family together. Jody became withdrawn and moody. She began to eat compulsively and put on weight. Her solace was a friend, whose parents were also divorced and who, like her, was also lacking the warmth and support of family life. The two girls began smoking cigarettes secretly when they were ten years old. At twelve they had their first experience of speed (amphetamines) and Jody was elated to discover how her confidence grew when she used this drug. Her appetite decreased and she lost weight. Finding a contact at school that guaranteed regular supply was no problem and she would use speed whenever she needed to face challenges at home, at school or meeting friends. She felt empowered, energised and liked her new-found assertiveness; she even began to enjoy her defiant behaviour. When she was fourteen she discovered tic (methamphetamine) whose action was much more powerful and longer lasting. She was introduced to a group of young drug users who would meet regularly to smoke tic through broken bottlenecks. The hangover gradually became so severe that she had to keep taking speed or smoking tic on her own to remove the intense discomfort. There was a rapid decline in her school progress, her health deteriorated and she had to begin pushing the drugs to finance her growing addiction. At age fifteen, when she started experimenting with cocaine, I was alerted that this girl had a problem and she was brought to me very reluctantly for her first consultation.

Cocaine (coke/snow/girl/lady)

I see your overpowerful will energising the body and especially the nervous system of all who are tempted by your power. Your high intelligence gives you the cunning and cleverness to attract your subjects and to conceal your presence.

—

Cocaine is one of the most addictive and dangerous of the illicit drugs. It is an alkaloid derived from the leaf of the cocoa plant (*Erythoxylon coca*) that native Americans chewed for thousands of years. It is an expensive drug, used mainly by affluent people, but increasingly used by all socio-economic groups. The white powder is inhaled (snorting – least dangerous), smoked or injected (freebasing – most dangerous), is felt almost immediately, and lasts only 30–60 minutes. Psychological dependence can develop after a single dose because of its personality-strengthening effects.

In the mid 1980s a much cheaper variation appeared on the world market. *Crack* is cocaine boiled with bicarbonate of soda which cools down and forms a sediment that can be broken into 'rocks' and smoked or injected. It has an extremely powerful and short-lived effect (3–5 minutes) causing extreme euphoria, overconfidence and aggression, and is highly addictive. While cocaine use is generally on the decline due to increased awareness of risks, crack use, especially among disadvantaged groups, is on the increase and is used most commonly by younger age groups. Nevertheless in the United Kingdom and USA, two to three percent of all people between the ages of 16–64 take cocaine.

Cocaine is taken primarily for its euphoria-producing and stimulating effects. The initial signs of stimulation are hyperactivity, restlessness, increased blood pressure, increased heart rate and euphoria. It is a drug that characteristically produces a heightened feeling of self-confidence, self-esteem, fearlessness and daring, giving users the euphoric perception of being capable of enhanced mental, intellectual, creative and physical achievements. It is most often used recreationally for this effect. This increased energy and power can quite easily develop into violent and emotional behaviour, exhibitionism and overstimulated sexual desire. This false sense of self pushes away feelings of insecurity, fears, doubts and pain which may explain why cocaine is an effective anaesthetic agent.[5]

Cocaine appears to block real human feelings, calling up instead icy-cold cynical thinking and feeling responses. The blocked expression of the heart mirrors the major pathological effects that are seen in the rhythmic organs of heart, circulation and respiration – increased heart and respiratory rate, hypertension, risk of heart attack, strokes, cardiac arrythmias, nasal and lung infections, respiratory and cardiac arrest. The soul forces are rearranged in the body; they move out of the sensory organs (anaesthetising effect) and the feeling/heart realm (blocked feelings) and engage deeply in the thinking and will activities of body and soul. The user becomes cut off from her higher spiritual nature and is thrust deeper into her lower material self where her intellect and her utilitarian nature become dominant, and frequently corrupted or distorted.

Amphetamines and related substances: speed/ice/crystal/crystal meth (tic)/CAT

You stand revealed as an extremely wilful, energising and physically empowering personality that imposes these powers on those that embrace you. Your deviousness is in the speed at which you work, which latches on to the will and bypasses the thinking.

These are chemical central nervous system stimulants with a drug profile very similar to those of cocaine but with a longer action (4–8 hours). They increase performance (used by athletes), induce euphoria and alertness and are used to combat exhaustion (students studying for exams, long-distance journeys). They are used therapeutically for a variety of clinical disorders including attention deficit disorder (administered as Ritalin), narcolepsy, depressive disorders and obesity. In Europe approximately 3% of the population between fifteen and sixty-four years of age have used amphetamines in their lifetime. Use of amphetamines appears to be on the increase worldwide. In South Africa, methamphetamine (tic) abuse has increased dramatically in all socio-economic groups, especially in certain regions where its use among the 12–17-year-old age group is at an alarmingly high level. Latest reports indicate that 10% of high school children in South Africa use tic.

Ritalin, also known as methylphenidate, is popular among high school and college students who use the medication to be able to stay alert and awake for long periods of time. There is a genuine potential for addiction to Ritalin if it is crushed and snorted, and when injected the effects are almost identical to cocaine. However, there is currently not sufficient evidence that methylphenidate is a suitable example of a cognitive enhancer with mass appeal.[6]

Methamphetamine (meth-tic-ice) can be inhaled, smoked or injected intravenously. Its psychological effects are powerful and last for hours. Unlike crack cocaine which must be imported, tic is a synthetic drug that can easily be manufactured locally. It produces an intense and long-lasting euphoria (24+ hours) and excitement followed by heavy hangover and depression which leads to rapid addiction. Withdrawal is characterised by excessive sleeping, eating and depression-like symptoms, often accompanied by anxiety and drug-craving.

Methcathinone (CAT) is also a scheduled psychoactive stimulant, sometimes used as a recreational drug and considered addictive. It is usually snorted but can be smoked, injected, or taken orally. The effects of methcathinone are similar to those of methamphetamine, initially regarded as less intense by the inexperienced user but often more euphoric.

Amphetamine-like substances that are cheap and easily available over the counter include *ephedrine* used for nasal congestion and *propranolamine* used as an appetite suppressant. Although less potent than classic amphetamines, they are potentially dangerous since three to four times the normal dose can lead to life-threatening hypertension, psychosis and death.

The stimulating and euphoric effects of these drugs, as with cocaine, induce the soul to engage more strongly with certain parts of the body, mainly the nervous system (increased cognitive activity) and the metabolic-will functions (enhanced stamina and power). In order for the body to regenerate its spent forces, the soul normally disengages with it during sleep which allows for restoration of vitality. This however does not happen when amphetamines are taken, leading to widespread and progressive breakdown and degeneration of the body. There is no space any longer for the user of amphetamines to embrace her higher self; she is forced to submit almost completely and permanently to the powers of the drug working through her soul and body.

Inhalants/solvents: benzene, petrol, glues, paint thinners

I see you as an earthly animalistic power that energises the blood with supernatural strength but then falls into slumber because you block the working of the brain.

—

These substances are inhaled, depress the central nervous system and produce effects similar to alcohol. They are usually used by children and adolescents who have ready access to these products. They are widely used by street kids as they help escape some of the realities of living on the streets, both on a social-psychological level (alienation, trauma, failed attachments) and a physical level (numbing cold weather).

The nature of these substances is to drive the soul further into the body. They force the user to bypass her higher self, her higher cognition and spirituality, confining her to the material world of earthly and sensuous pleasures.

Cosmic drugs

Tembi grew up in an informal settlement outside Cape Town. Her mother was a domestic worker, her father worked in a factory. Her parents left for work in the early morning and came home after dark, and as an early child she was looked after by neighbours. She was sexually molested on several occasions by unemployed men who lay around the neighbourhood. She was a timid and reserved girl in junior school with few friends and then when her father was killed in a factory accident, she retreated into a dream world of her own. A year later when Tembi was nine years old, her mother's boyfriend moved in to their small shack. She had to endure several years of sexual abuse and was raped frequently when her mother was away. Her way of coping with these traumatic experiences was to block off all thoughts and feelings relating to the abuse. She began to smoke marijuana when she was twelve and found deep comfort and relief from the tensions and anxieties of her life. Marijuana became her way of escaping from these harsh and painful realities, at the cost of cutting herself off from all experiences that were uncomfortable for her.

I heard about Tembi's case from a fellow counsellor when she was sixteen years old, one of thousands of such adolescents in my area who receive no help and whose lives and personalities degenerate under the excruciating burden of living with these dangerous substances. If nothing were done to help her and children like her, it is likely she would habitually learn to avoid, deny and withdraw herself from all difficult and uncomfortable situations, relying always on the assistance of outside agents or behaviour patterns to gratify her need for safety. She would never consciously take responsibility for herself.

Cannabis: marijuana (grass, weed, pot, dagga, ganga), hashish (resin of cannabis buds)

You come from a world of fine sensing and feeling luring your subjects into this world of beauty and heightened imagination with your soft and relaxed nature. You will not tolerate the fixed patterns of earthly reality, casting it aside with disinterest and disdain and creating a way of being that brings peace and calmness. When the earthly life however intrudes itself too powerfully, you may well bring fear and doubt to those you have enslaved.

Cannabis is a genus of flowering plants that includes three putative species, *Cannabis sativa*, *Cannabis indica*, and *Cannabis ruderalis*, and is probably the most widely used illicit drug in the world. It is estimated that about 4% of the world's adult population use cannabis annually. In 1995, 77% of illicit drug users were using marijuana or hashish. In the past decade the rate of use among adolescents has more than doubled and the age of first use is becoming younger (8–9 years). It has psychoactive and physiological effects when consumed, usually by smoking or ingestion which will vary according to factors such as potency, dose, chemical composition, method of consumption mind set and setting. The cannabis user may be transported for several hours by the power of this drug into a reality where she perceives things from a higher vantage point (feeling high), loses contact with accustomed earthly realities and enters a world of heightened sensitivity and intensified feelings. This opens up vivid imaginative experiences rich with inner personal meaning and the release of intense emotions, for instance, overwhelming love for the world, religious experiences of the divine in all things, or negative emotional experiences such as fear and suspicion. Higher doses can lead to distortions of objects and even hallucinations. This heart-knowing is at the expense of sober logical head-knowing, becoming more disassociative, expansive, creative and free of earthly restraints. Indeed many young people who use cannabis reject the materialistic western way of thinking, seeking a return to nature, community living, ecological awareness and eastern spirituality. They join together in close feeling bonds and deep friendships to the exclusion of non-users. The 'joint', the cannabis cigarette that is handed around in a group, becomes a symbol of joining together with other like-minded individuals who are striving for similar values. Cannabis lifts the soul and self out of the body, leading to a waking-dreaming consciousness; the physical body then becomes part of the outer world, feels heavy like a stone (feeling stoned), and becomes more difficult to use (will weakness).

Hallucinogenic/psychedelic drugs

There are more than one hundred known natural and synthetic substances that induce a loss of contact with normal earthly reality, heightened consciousness and hallucinations. The most well-known naturally occurring hallucinogens are certain mushrooms (psilocybin or magic mushrooms), psilocybin derived from these mushrooms, and mescaline derived from the peyote cactus. The classic synthetic hallucinogen is LSD (lysergic acid diethylamide) derived from the parasitic fungus ergot that grows on and destroys the flowering part of the rye cereal.

Lysergic acid diethylamide (LSD)

You are a divine wizard with supersensible access to cosmic realms. You have the power to magically transform your subjects into apprentice wizards who, for a short while, are able to gaze into the cosmic world that lives behind earthly reality.

—

Lysergic acid diethylamide, LSD-25, or acid, is a semisynthetic psychedelic drug considered mainly as a recreational drug – an *entheogen* – and as a means for transcendence. Once ingested, a normal dose takes effect within an hour, peaks in 2–4 hours, and lasts 8–12 hours. Sensory perceptions become unusually intense, vivid and more conscious as the soul separates from the body; colours are richer and more brilliant, shapes and textures are more striking, tastes and smells are intensified, and sounds are magnified. The user can be transported through outer sense impressions or through inner imaginative pictures into highly evocative experiences that may or may not relate to what she has experienced previously in her life. Sense impressions flow one into another (synaesthesia) – colours may be heard and music seen. The life body (*prana, chi,* etheric body) that prevents the living body from physically disintegrating (death) also loosens itself from the physical body, producing short-lived experiences of near-death. Descriptions of thousands of LSD experiences are very similar to the cases documented by Raymond Moody and Elizabeth Kubler-Ross of individuals who appeared to have died or who almost died. Violent shocks are known to separate the life body from the physical body; the former fuses with the soul life so that its memory content comes to awareness in soul imagery. A typical experience is the life panorama where flashbacks to life events, for instance prenatal or postnatal, come to consciousness in a very vivid way. Repressed or forgotten memories of past traumas, for instance concentration camp syndrome, may be powerfully re-evoked. The dissolution of inner and outer boundaries, with the feeling of blissful light-filled oneness with everything, is a common experience as the life forces merge with their cosmic origin. Alterations in body shape, distortions of time and space, awareness of internal organs and functions as well as visions and hallucinations may also occur, all as if in a waking dream. Intense emotional, religious and mystical experiences accompanied by deep inner reflection are common. Many users claim that significant personality changes such as enhanced creative capacities, deep insights, and relief from neurotic and psychosomatic symptoms have taken place through a single LSD experience.[7]

The effects on the user will depend on their emotional and mental state, psychological history, previous experiences, environmental setting, degree of psychological resilience or vulnerability, and of course the amount of substance used.

Psilocybin mushrooms

These are fungi that contain the psychedelic substances psilocybin and psilocin. They are also called magic mushrooms or 'shrooms. The intoxicating effects typically last from three to seven hours depending on amount ingested, the strength of the plant, the method of preparation and individual metabolism. The experience is usually oriented inwardly, with powerful visual, auditory and revelationary components and may be exhilarating or distressing. One may experience the withdrawal of one's lower self and the emergence of a higher or cosmic awareness. There may also be a total absence of effects, even with large doses.

Opiates-opioids: opium, morphine, heroin

The words 'opiate' and 'opioid' derive from the word 'opium', the milk sap of the opium poppy, *Papaver somniferum* , which is extracted by cutting open the capsule of the plant. Opium has gradually been superseded by a variety of purified, semi-synthetic and synthetic opioids with progressively stronger effects than the unripe capsule of the plant. Opium contains approximately twenty opium alkaloids, including morphine. Opiates are any preparation or derivative of opium (morphine, heroin, codeine); opioids are synthetic narcotics that resemble an opiate in action but are not derived from opium (wellconal, pethidine, methadone, demerol). Because codeine-containing painkillers are readily accessible over the counter, they are widely abused and frequently lead to addictive dependencies. Because of their easy accessibility over the counter, painkillers with codeine are widely abused as well. In Europe approximately 0.1–0.6% of the population use opiates. All these narcotic drugs have similar effects but because heroin is the most commonly used narcotic in young people it will be described below.

Heroin – H

You are revealed as a divine goddess living in bliss and ecstacy, with the power to evoke in your subjects the most ecstatic and euphoric feelings and sensations.

—

Heroin is synthesised from morphine but is about twice as potent. Users typically start in their teens, even as young as ten years old, and usually in communities where substance abuse is rampant. Fifty percent of urban heroin users are children of single parents or divorced parents, and are from families in which at least one other member has a substance-related disorder. Prevalence varies greatly from country to country and changes from year to year. In South Africa increasingly younger people are starting to use heroin and for most of these users, heroin is their first drug of choice. Peter, a young patient of mine, was thirteen years when he was admitted to a psychiatric clinic. Heroin is so addictive because of the overwhelming euphoric high (rush or flash) that occurs, especially when administered intravenously. However, as the risk of contracting HIV escalated, the user pattern has changed from intravenous to inhaling it – 'chasing the dragon'. Most people who currently present with heroin dependence are smokers not IV users, although there are many who progress from 'chasing' to 'spiking'.

After crossing the blood-brain barrier it converts into morphine which mimics the action of the endorphins, creating a heightened sense of wellbeing. This euphoria feeling has been described as an 'orgasm' centred in the gut.

This drug, like all the opium-related substances, seems to belong to a world beyond the earthly plane. It produces in the user an almost immediate expansive blissful feeling of warmth associated with deep relaxation and peace which frees her of all tensions, worries and cares (the life forces separate from the physical body); she can completely escape into a light floating world where she is totally alone with her heroin Goddess, her great lover, losing almost all connection with body and soul. Heroin's fire powerfully drives the self out of body and soul. The user remains only connected to her thinking, which becomes cold, distant and calculating; fear is driven away. Gradually she becomes quiet, soft and tender, anaesthetised from all pain, passing into a dreamy sleepy state. The soul separates from the body (release from pain, fear and consciousness). The euphoria and sedation are soon replaced by the fear of withdrawal accompanied by emptiness and depression that drives the user to find her next fix. She becomes completely controlled by the 4–6-hour rhythm of opiates in her blood, to the exclusion of all other needs. Her physical and psychological condition deteriorates. Heroin loosens the user from earthly realities.

Mandrax: methaqualone, buttons, mx, whites, pille

This minor tranquilliser is smoked widely in South Africa, together with cannabis in a broken bottleneck. Between 70 and 80% of the global use of mandrax takes place in South Africa. As the soul separates from the body intense euphoria, heightened perceptions and sensations and reduced inhibitions occur.

Earthly and cosmic drugs

There are some drugs that manifest both earthly and cosmic attributes:

Modified amphetamines

These include Ecstasy (E, pills, MDMA, XTC, Adam, hug drug, smarties), MDEA (Eve) and STP (DOM), of which Ecstasy is the most widely available and best studied.

Ecstasy

You are surely a being of great diversity carrying both the power of the earth and the wisdom of the heart. Those who use you are filled with your physical strength and blessed with your power of love and compassion.

—

This substance, originally derived from nutmeg oil, was synthesised in the 1960s and used in the 1970s psychotherapeutically to help patients get in touch with their feelings. Since the 1980s its recreational use has increased dramatically. It has become popular with young people at parties, raves and clubs where it promotes warm feelings and increased stamina for dancing, as well as with affluent and professional people in social and communal get-togethers where it engenders openness,

115

euphoria, love, happiness and mental clarity. Tactile sensations are enhanced for some users, making physical contact with others more pleasurable and expressive. Ecstasy combines the hallucinogenic effects of cannabis/LSD with the stimulant effects of amphetamines. It is classed as a hallucinogenic amphetamine. Its nature draws power from both earthly and cosmic realms, forcing the user to engage with both realities, offering the allure of a truly holistic and unified experience of self. One part of the soul seems to separate from the body, leading to an expansion of consciousness with tremendously heightened sensory and feeling experience – feeling free, relaxed and deeply at peace with the world and oneself, dissolving in euphoric oneness with a highly luminescent world and fusing in blissful loving warm union with other people. At the same time, another aspect of the soul connects powerfully with the body leading to a desire for movement, dancing or other actions or for company, conversation or personal interaction.

The drug usually enters awareness within half an hour, lasts three to six hours followed by a gradual comedown. It has an effect on the body's internal thermostat resulting in dangerous overheating and dehydration in hot places where the user dances for long periods. It can also lead to urinary retention so that sudden drinking of large quantities of fluids can cause dangerous fluid and salt imbalance. People predisposed to heart and blood pressure conditions, asthma and epilepsy may experience serious adverse effects. There have been over two hundred Ecstasy-related deaths in the UK since 1996.

Designer drugs (substituted amphetamines)

These are fairly recent drug creations designed on the drawing board to manipulate consciousness in a variety of different ways (earthly or cosmic). Most begin as legal substances that are modified slightly to produce a specifically desired alteration in consciousness. By the time they have been researched, found to be harmful and banned as illegal drugs, they have already found a wide clientele; through their cheap and simple manufacture in clandestine laboratories they are widely distributed through drug cartels. These substances are extremely potent, with small quantities producing extremely powerful effects.

What are the dangers for young people becoming addicted to illicit drugs?

This is a subject that could fill many books and there is a library of literature that details the general risks and dangers of these drugs, as well as the harmful effects of specific drugs.[5,7,8] The description of the individual drug substances listed above outline some of these effects.

Apart from the physical and psychological effects there are of course a wide range of psycho-developmental, social and educational outcomes that result from drug addiction. The young person becomes trapped in a cycle of dependency that can completely disrupt her normal psycho-social development. Most of us will have heard, or know about, heart wrenching cases of children or young adults who have become caught up in the destructive spiral of drug addiction which has devastated their young lives.

Miranda was an adopted child, molested and abused by her adoptive parents. She started smoking tic when she was thirteen years of age, becoming defiant and anti-social and began socialising with drug minded youth. When she was not using the drug she was constantly tired and moody; she was always fighting with her parents, lost her best friends and fell behind in school. At fifteen she was using heroin, she dropped out of school and left home with her boyfriend. She started selling her body to pay for her drugs, was caught in possession of heroin and spent time in a juvenile detention centre. She became pregnant at sixteen, took an overdose and was admitted to a rehabilitation centre where she managed finally, after many months, to come clean.

Drug-dependent youth are exposed to greater risks of accidents of all kinds, injury, violence, unsafe sex, unwanted pregnancies, suicide and contracting infectious diseases such as HIV/AIDS, hepatitis and tuberculosis; they are at risk of being charged with illegal possession or drug dealing, going to jail and receiving a criminal record; of becoming caught up in unsavoury associations with drug dealers and other addicts; of dropping out of school or college and compromising their future careers, of causing the breakdown in relationships and untold misery and grief to themselves and their family. And while they are in the grips of dependency they may have to face an intellectual, emotional and moral decline that can scar them for life. But perhaps the greatest risk and danger is becoming enslaved to the drug lord itself who takes control of the young person's body, soul and spirit, demanding that she gives up her freedom and in so doing loses contact with her higher self.

Drugs as one-sided pathology

Health may be seen as the balance between heaven and earth, between cosmic-spiritual and earthly-material forces, and ill health as a disturbance of this relationship. If the tendency towards hardening, mineralisation, contraction, drying out and cooling down is balanced out by processes that create softening, dissolution, expansion, moisturising and warming, then homeostasis is maintained. Organic systems are so constructed that when too much contraction occurs, for instance when a muscle goes into spasm, regulative processes kick in that lead to expansion – in this case, the muscle relaxes. When a child's body cools down to a certain degree, fever results that leads to a resetting of the body's thermostat. In nature there are substances that are governed more by earthly forces (earth, water), others more by cosmic forces (air, light, warmth). The illicit drugs are all powerful one-sided substances that possess either one or other (or both) tendencies. As such they are the antithesis of healthy substances; they are instruments of disease tendencies, carrying forces that promote one-sided tendencies. These drugs are highly dangerous to all children before and after puberty for the reasons mentioned in the previous chapter. Furthermore those children who have tendencies in one or other direction (earthly or cosmic) will be especially vulnerable to the effects of these drugs.

Helping youngsters addicted to illicit substances

How can we help teenagers and adolescents who have succumbed to the seductive effects of drugs?

The approach for drug addiction is essentially the same as that put forward in earlier chapters with certain modifications.

Once again we will need to understand the nature of drug dependency and addiction and see it as a cry for help. The child is in deep need of something she is missing and the drug, as the false saviour, becomes the refuge and the diversion for the vulnerability and the inner needs that have not been met. With this as our starting point, we apply the same method and application as outlined in Chapter 2 to deepen our understanding of addiction and the child who is addicted.

Our first duty to the child in need is to check our attitudes to ourselves and to the child who is misusing the drug. This requires honest self-reflection about our values, prejudices and position especially towards dependency, addiction and illicit substances, as well as about the way they are expressed in our behaviour and parenting. Can we expect our children to adopt healthy values when we ourselves cannot carry them out? 'Why should I stop smoking and drinking when I see my parents doing the same?' We shall get nowhere if we hold on to old preconceptions, denial, guilt, fear, or lecturing about drugs.

Once we have cleared our own inner state of mind, we can focus on the child. However, we can only begin to understand the child if we open ourselves to her with sufficient interest and respect. Accepting her for who she is and meeting her needs as her truth and her reality, is the surest way of gaining her trust. Through our general understanding of the road map of child development, we are able to see where she has arrived on this journey.

We proceed to develop a broad picture experience of the child through the observational method described, entering more and more deeply into the child's experience through our own experiential involvement. An understanding of the child's profile will help us to understand the needs and expressions of this unique child in her specific stage of development. To this we add also our understanding of the child's specific temperament and character, and we try to see the child in the context of her environment. A clear picture of the child's home, school and social environment will assist in assessing either what is missing in the child's life, or what is contributing to the drug dependency. The home environment is usually the first place where the child or adolescent expects to find understanding, safety and support. Every effort will need to be made to create the most optimal home conditions possible.

We will also need to assess the degree of the child's addictive behaviour. Parents must be able to detect warning signs of substance misuse or abuse (chronic tiredness; unusual eye symptoms such as red eyes, dilated or constricted pupils; changes in appetite and sleep patterns; sudden shifts in emotions and moods; fall-off in performance and loss of motivation and interest). One requires some idea of the seriousness of the drug habit: is it youthful exploration, peer pressure, a strong dependency or full-on addiction. When and where does it take place?

We shall invariably discover, when we endeavour to experience inwardly the core issue of drug addiction, that the drug satisfies temporarily the deeper need of the user by removing the pain and discomfort caused by the neediness (see box).

Unfulfilled primary need → pain → blocking of the need → ensuing discomfort → the finding and adopting of a substitute gratification → appeases the pain briefly → secondary need → dependency on substitute agency

There are some drug addicts who appear to have no deep seated missing needs: they have been well cared for as children, supported through school, and have no apparent behaviour problems. They come into contact with the drug and within a short time have become dependent on it. These are individuals whose addiction is frequently not based on pain that must be blocked, but rather on pleasure that cannot be resisted. They are usually youth that are highly sensitive, impressionable and too open to the world in which they live. They lack the power of self to resist the gratuitous pleasures brought to them by the drug. In these cases, however, we still find that the dependency develops on the basis of some innate factor that is missing – in this case *self-control*.[8]

With clear understanding of both the addictive phenomenon and this addicted child, we can move forward towards helping the child. This will of course depend on whether the child wants to be helped. It is essential that some kind of meaningful partnership is established and for this to occur, an effective communication with the child needs to follow, aimed at engaging the higher truth and conscience of the child. The conditions and guidelines for enhancing communication are described in detail in Chapter 3. Only on the basis of mutual trust and respect can new insights, accurate assessment and clear perspectives for effective care and management follow.

Having created a partnership with the dependent client, it may be helpful to try to involve family members, schoolteachers and community members in the therapeutic team. They can provide the containing structure that the client needs for her rehabilitation and welcoming return to healthy community life. However, this requires the co-operation and motivation of the young client, and needs always to be negotiated on an individual basis with the client herself.

Once commitment and motivation to overcoming the addiction has been achieved, a written contract based on accountability and time frames needs to be made. On this basis the clinical management of the case should be constructed. This will include a clinical assessment and the design of a therapeutic programme.

In my view, a holistic multi-dimensional contractual therapeutic programme involving the young client, her parents, teachers, community members, health practitioner and therapists, offers a rational and effective approach to drug addiction and addictive tendencies. Once the health status of the client has been assessed clinically and biochemically, an appropriate detox programme should be instituted using dietary and nutritional interventions, individually-prescribed natural and dynamic medication, and intravenous infusions aimed at supporting weakened organ systems and the elimination of toxic substances.

A wide range of therapeutic interventions, aimed at meeting individual dispositions and working with the individual client, can actively support the rehabilitation process. These include movement therapies (eurythmy, dancing, Bothmer gymnastics, Kung Fu), art therapies (painting, clay modelling, drawing), craft therapies (woodwork, iron forging, weaving, leather work, jewellery, canework) and working with nature (gardening, farm work, caring for animals, equine assisted therapy – hippotherapy). Research into these different therapies, their specific character and connection to the human constitution is the subject of a work in process.[9]

Counselling is an essential part of the therapeutic and rehabilitative process. I have found psychophonetic counselling and coaching to be especially effective in dealing with drug addiction.

In severe cases of drug dependency, in situations where the client is in danger of self-harm or when there is serious clinical decompensation, referral to specialist care and rehabilitation centres may be unavoidable.

Jody denied she had a drug problem. Because this was clearly a symptom of a deeper lying problem, nothing was said about this problem for the first few sessions. Interest, respect and trust in the child's life destiny had first to be found if we were to get anywhere.

Behind the initial resistance and the pseudo-assertive stance she took, was a vulnerable sensitive girl who was warmed by the interest someone took in her background. We were then able to enter deeply into her background, her family life and inner experiences. Trust gradually grew between us until she was able to speak freely about her drug addiction. Step by step, she developed insight and a clear perspective of the problem and she was finally able to make a choice to break out of the stranglehold the drugs had on her. This threshold was the turning point in her journey to overcome her addiction. She understood that on the one hand she had to take care of the vulnerable anxious girl inside of her who was in deep need of support; on the other that she had to find the strength to withstand the powerful temptations of taking substances she knew would immediately take away her pain and discomfort. We knew she needed support for this work and so together with her mother, a schoolteacher, an art therapist and masseur, we constructed together a programme to which she could fully commit. She embarked on a six week programme that included regular intravenous detox infusions, oral vitamins, mineral, herbal and homeopathic supplementation, diet therapy, art therapy, massage therapy and psychophonetic counselling-coaching sessions.

Jody had to make contact on a daily basis with that vulnerable part inside her that used the drugs, to satisfy her deep need for care and support. She learnt to meet this place inside of her by sensing the bodily sensations that arose when she remembered or felt her helplessness and anxiety and then creating the appropriate physical gesture that corresponded with this bodily awareness. By moving away from the place where she performed the gesture, she was able to visualise the frightened girl within her, the way it was living unseen inside of her. This way she could directly meet this part of herself. She then learned exactly what was needed to support and care for her, either a confident reassuring loving mother or father, or friend or mentor. She would then resource within herself this supportive character by inwardly feeling this person, sensing and transforming her bodily stature, just like an actress playing the chosen role in a drama. In this role, she would now actively do something to demonstrate her loving support for the vulnerable child.

But she also learned to recognise the power each particular drug had over her; she would enter the nature of tic, taking on the power of this drug as it affected her vulnerable nature. It was as if she became and acted out the being of the substance, then stood aside and saw it for what it was and how it acted on her vulnerability. She discovered that what was needed to counter its action was resourcing the very counter power within her that could confront and remove the seductive power of the drug. This always took the form of a calm, confident, strong and loving personality, always protective in its nature.

Regular practice and vigilant attention to her inner feelings and bodily sensations enabled Jody to overcome her addiction and take personal responsibility for her own emotional needs. She will need to be constantly aware of her dispositions in order to maintain her healthy equilibrium.

Tembi is highly unlikely to seek help herself, nor is it likely that her mother, family members or teachers would even realise she has a problem. Her world is closed off to almost everyone. Does one have to wait for her problem to escalate to life threatening proportions before something is done to help her and when it is so much more difficult to repair the damage? Her issue is also a social and educational one. The drug is her answer to the lack of parental and educational awareness and care. For if someone had been aware of Tembi's plight early on, measures could be put in place to protect her. It is of course wishful thinking, to imagine the necessary social structures that would need to be in place for the disadvantaged populace. Most often these children and adolescents are left on their own to find ways of surviving the most heinous circumstances. And they do cope, usually at great cost to themselves and to society at large. It is their great fortune to meet someone who is willing to take on the responsibility of helping them find their own self-respect, self-worth and self-care.

Illicit drugs may be regarded as agents of two cultural forces in our times that coercively and unnaturally either pull vulnerable youth more into their bodies (material dominance) or push them out of their bodies (spiritual dominance). In both cases they subvert the guiding power of the developing child that can make choices and free decisions. Young people easily succumb to the temptation of these substances because of their vulnerability and unconscious longing to satisfy unfulfilled needs. Furthermore, children with drug dependencies are invariably sensitive individuals who have the specific one-sided tendencies mentioned above (earthly, cosmic). These seductive substances, like false prophets, may take control of young bodies and souls, creating unimaginable chaos and destruction in their lives and in the lives of those who care for them. However, they may also serve as messengers revealing the human potential that every young person is capable of reaching through his or her own efforts.

Chapter 7. The Tyranny of the Entertainment Media

I give the TV in my living room many meanings. It is a messenger of the world, a well-informed communicator, a fabulous entertainer and an excellent relaxer. But it is also an intruder in the home, a disturber of the peace, a thief of creativity and a tyrant that binds the soul. It speaks a language that enthrals the mind and captivates desire. Children and youth are especially at the mercy of its seductive nature. If we are to protect our children from the fascinating power of the entertainment media, we need to understand what it is and how to tame it.

—

For large sections of society, television has become the dominating symbol of modern life.[1] Most people can do without a radio, but not a TV. It is the world in your living room and an answer to many needs. It is excellent company, it gives pleasure and comfort. It can make one feel worldly informed and locally connected, empowered as a global citizen, and it is highly entertaining; for whenever one chooses, in the comfort of one's home and at the press of a button, one has access to a selection of home entertainment. Even the poorest can feel they are part of the bigger world, participating in their fantasy with sensational stories of other people's lives. For most children and adolescents it has become an indispensable part of life.

Yet while it connects and empowers outwardly, inwardly it can quite easily disconnect and disempower people from their own self, leading to dependency and addiction. And children and youth more than any other section of society are at risk of losing their innocence, their innate creativity and their connection to reality through an authoritarian control by the entertainment media where TV, after many decades, still stands at centre stage.

Although this chapter includes the other entertainment media, such as cinema, home movies, videos and DVDs, the focus here will be on the

TV since, by the very position that it occupies in the child's life, it offers itself more than the others as an addictive agency.

Why do you watch TV and how does it make you feel?

I choose to switch on the television, watch a DVD or go to the movies, for one of several reasons. I may be wanting to relax, switch off and escape into a world where I have very little to do except passively watch the changing images on the screen. I notice how tired this escapism makes me. Or I am looking to be entertained by professional entertainers and a sophisticated entertainment medium that provide me with a sensational, externally-stimulated creative experience that gives me pleasure, comfort and satisfaction. I am aware I have myself not created this fantasy world that excites, humours, delights, terrorises, horrifies or depresses me. I also notice that unless I make a conscious effort to oppose it, I can quite easily be tempted to want more of it. Or, I am wishing to be informed about something that interests me – the news, a speech, an event, or documentary. Here I feel I am more in control of my thinking regarding the subject matter and can enter inwardly or externally into discourse with the information presented.

Recall how children and teenagers watch TV. Most young children who enter a room with the TV on will be immediately fascinated and captivated by the sounds and images on the screen and it is difficult to draw their attention away from the screen. Even the adult eye and ear is automatically drawn there and it needs an effort of will to control the roving eye. Children, who in their early years live so strongly in the world of senses, cannot do this unless they have other more interesting objects to distract them. TV, with its short sound bites and rapid firing picture images, is specifically designed to capture the viewer's attention. Teenagers who are bored and have nothing better to do will tend to slouch on the sofa and watch whatever is on the screen without discernment, sometimes for hours on end, perhaps switching from one programme to the other. Those who are more inwardly disciplined or have other interests can curtail the time spent viewing. Others who have less self-control are caught up in this world of make believe. A significant portion of these youth will become dependent and even addicted to it, fulfilling criteria used clinically to define substance abuse: they spend a great deal of time watching TV and more time than they intend; they may think about reducing it or make unsuccessful attempts to do so; it becomes repetitive, compulsive and they give up important social or other occupational activities to use it and continue to do so despite harmful consequences; they experience withdrawal symptoms when stopping its use.

The addiction phenomenon

We are witnessing throughout the developed and developing world an ever-growing body-mind dependency of children and youth to some substance or activity. At the core of all dependency and addiction, there will invariably be found real needs that have not been fully satisfied. This leads to the search and the adoption of a substitutive answer to appease the pain of these unfulfilled needs. An addictive partnership is thereby established between a compelling force that provides gratification and the needy person who becomes captive to this gratification. One of these compelling forces in the culture of our times is the entertainment media.

Children and youth with unsatisfied needs, who in their phase of development lack the ability to protect themselves from such forces, can easily become dependent on this compelling force.

Historical perspectives

Between 1940 and 1950, the electric and graphic revolution came together in the development of television and by 1950 had become well entrenched in American homes. TV only came to South Africa in 1976 and at that time addictive behaviour in childhood and adolescence was much less common than it is today. One can well ask what role TV has played in the development of this cultural phenomenon.

Civilisations are shaped by the means of communication between people. First there was the oral word which developed into language, then came pictographic signs such as hieroglyphics and later the abstract alphabet that enabled language to be written down and read. The printing press in the middle of the fifteenth century radically changed the face of human communication. Communication moved from the ear to the eye and the first mass medium was created for every branch of life. The revolutionary discovery by Samuel Morse in 1832 of the electric telegraph, whereby information could be transmitted electrically and independently of time, space and person, heralded the birth of electronic communication. The news industry was created. Between 1850 and 1950 communication was further modified by the inventions of photography, the telephone, the phonograph, the gramophone, cinema, radio and finally television. The picture took over from the word as the dominant means of mass communication.[2]

The rise of the TV genie

The TV genie is well and truly out of the box and has become a partner in the life of most people and an active member of most families. In the USA, 99% of children have a TV set in their homes; one third of children from babies up to six years of age live in homes where the TV is on almost all the time; 70% of eight to eighteen year olds have a set in their bedrooms; 50% of homes have three or more TV sets; 80% of children younger than age six watch TV, play video games or use the computer on average for two hours daily; 95% live in homes with at least one DVD player. The average child watches four hours of TV daily.[3]

Statistics about TV are moving in this direction in all developed and developing countries.[4,5,6]

The nature of the TV genie

One may well ask what is the nature of this force that fosters this addictive behaviour and compels many children and teenagers to spend more time watching TV than all other activities, apart from school life and sleeping?

Most of us have experienced this compelling force. Simply recall how the TV screen holds your attention so powerfully. Yet television is only compelling because the viewer finds it compelling. If, one fine day, everyone were to find TV banal and boring, this medium would quickly disappear into the archives of technological history. We switch off the TV when we no longer find it interesting. TV only exists because some part of the human psyche wants it to exist, wants what it provides, and finds pleasure in what it offers. Some clever social scientists and psychologists have recognised the needs of this part of the human psyche and, together with highly creative programme designers, have discovered ingenious ways of making a connection with the psyche and holding its attention. For it is the magical power of this medium to hold the attention of the viewer so completely, that keeps the psyche spellbound. Here are some of the ways it does this:

- All programmes, whether they are news broadcasts, documentaries, shows of all kinds, sporting events, educational, religious or political presentations, are arranged in the form of entertainment, narratives and story lines. Who of us do not enjoy being entertained?
- The sensory encounter is highly stimulating, alluring and engaging: this is achieved by providing prominent foreground visual stimulation in the form of dynamic, exquisitely crafted and beautifully photographed, constantly changing visual images of short duration (on average 3.5 seconds), visual and auditory startle effects, underpinned with background emotive music that creates the right atmosphere, appropriate voice narrative and loud sound grabs that wake one up at the right moment. We dare not let our attention waver lest we miss something!
- The programme content is designed for maximum and continuous sensation-grabbing, novelty and interest aimed at fascination, excitement, arousal and the latest sensational disclosures. This will keep us on the edge of our seat, and ... what might we hear next!
- The viewer is constantly offered things that he aspires to, longs for, likes and desires, aimed solely at emotional gratification: I am held in the 'maybe one day' fantasy, if only I could drive that car or become famous like him, or if I can't play cricket like him, at least I can watch and support him.
- Psychological activities that require serious mental or intellectual activity such as sophisticated adult judgment, rational and analytical skills, are mostly avoided. No time is given between shots to reflect on what was seen or heard. When we need to relax and escape from the hardships of life, the last thing we want to do is to think! These are aspects commonly associated with the addictive process.
- Since the TV usually occupies a central place in the home,

it cannot easily be hidden and requires minimal skills to operate; all programmes are accessible to anyone able to press a button. This way, as many of us as possible are part of the game.[7]

The other side of the partnership is, of course, that part of the human soul that needs this nourishment and devours the food provided. What is its nature?

We have seen that the soul or psyche is that inner experience which provides the human being with an inner life, made up of sensitivity, feeling, thinking and will impulses such as drives and desires. The entertainment media, working like an active compelling partner, engages with and stimulates certain aspects of the human psyche that behaves like a passive, submissive partner. It latches on to the sensing soul that sees and hears, the will that desires and craves for sensation and stimulation and the feelings that are played on passively like a musical instrument. The activity of thinking is used only to cognise and give meaning to what has been perceived and experienced. Compare the soul activity of a child watching TV with one playing in a garden, where the senses of movement, balance, life, touch, smell, taste and others are also actively involved; or with one reading an intriguing book where the child's active and personal creative imagination, inspired by the story line is replaced in watching TV by the visual and auditory images that the child is compelled to absorb passively from the outside. In reading, through his own mental picture building, his feelings and ideas, the child creates his own experience of the characters in the book, what the environment looks like etc. It is well established that for many children, television has replaced or curtailed reading other than magazines or comic books.

John was only six months old when he was introduced to TV because it was a convenient way of keeping a very active child occupied. His parents were so proud that he could remain attentive for such long periods. They did not realise that his attention deficit and hyperactivity, that became apparent in nursery school, could have well been worsened by TV viewing. TV then became a means of containing his exuberance and helping him to concentrate better. However, the exact opposite seemed to be the case. In his first year of primary school, he was the most disruptive and inattentive child in the class. His behaviour was always worse after watching TV the night before school. He could not apply himself to learning to write and read or to listening to the teacher without interrupting, and exhibited no imaginative capacities. His behaviour became so bad that the principal demanded that he be put on Ritalin or find another school.

Children and youth who become dependent on TV and other entertainment media have an overwhelming need to be entertained, stimulated and excited by the fantasy life of show business because their real life is either too boring or too uncomfortable. In both cases they are unhappy with who, what and where they are, and mostly doing their best to get away from themselves. We may recall the earthly-cosmic disposition referred to in previous chapters. TV reinforces the tendency that would draw us away from the earth and our own physical bodies, allowing us to become more spiritual, artistic, creative, desiring, sensuous and wilful, and seeking out sensation and excitement. A troubled cosmic child who lives more strongly in her soul and spirit would naturally and effortlessly be drawn into this illusory world of make believe. On the other hand, an unhappy earthly child who lives more strongly in his body would enjoy the opportunity to get away from his body as often as possible. The entertainment media is the perfect nourishment to satisfy this longing to be free of the heaviness of life.

The effects of TV

At this point we must ask the inevitable question: what is the effect of TV on our children and youth? How harmful is it really, especially for those who watch for hours every day or are addicted to TV? And are there any positive benefits?

These questions are relevant for many people at the present time as a cursory search on the internet on Google rendered millions of articles on the effects of TV on brain development alone. In this book it is not possible to review this huge and controversial subject in a comprehensive manner. There are a multitude of serious studies that point towards the damaging effects of TV and other electronic entertainment media on the physical, psychological, mental, social and educational health of children and adolescents. There are other studies that discount or underplay the damage. Will we risk the health of our children by ignoring the potential risks or adopting a wait-and-see attitude? Do we have to wait for so called health authorities to tell us that entertainment media are good or bad for our children? Can we be alert to the research that is out there and use our own experience and healthy judgment in deciding what effects are likely to be true and to what extent we will allow our children and youth to be exposed to the entertainment media?

With training in self-reflection and mindfulness, one can observe the effects that TV has on one's own soul functions. One may notice how the TV images and sound impressions impact on one's audio-visual perceptions and affect one's body functions, feelings, emotions and will capacities (drives, desires, motivations, wishes, resolutions) in specific ways. For instance, one may observe how the images of a coffee commercial may stimulate the taste and smell of coffee, start digestive juices secreting, set off the desire and need for coffee and push one to go and make a cup of coffee. One can also live into the experience of the child glued to the TV in the way described methodologically in this book. Using such guided experience together with the ever-increasing research into this topic, one can determine the likely effects on the three principal systems of the human constitution.[8-14]

Neuro-sensory system and cognitive functions

Although research dealing with effects of the media on early brain development is still in its infancy, neuroscientists have clearly established that environmental experiences significantly shape the developing brain due to the plasticity of the young unformed nerve tissue. Close contact with loving care-givers and the natural elemental world will have a different effect on neuro-sensory development. *The American Academy of Paediatrics has recommended since 1999 that children under the age of two years should not watch TV because it 'can negatively affect early brain development.'*[9] A study of 2,500 children in *Paedriatrics*, the journal of the AAP, concluded that children who watch TV up to three years of age have a significantly increased risk of developing attentional problems by age seven. There is a 9% increase in attentional damage for every hour watched. Attention deficit disorder, with or without hyperactivity, is the most common and fastest growing childhood disorder in the developed world.[10] TV viewing increases slower alpha brain waves associated with decreased mental activity, trance dreamlike states and increased dopamine levels [11,14]

TV and computer viewing have been blamed for a rising incidence of myopia and other eye damage. Every image on the screen is a mosaic of light points produced by the cathode ray of the TV and which fly across the screen through half a million image points in 1/30th of a second and then start again from the beginning. The complete mosaic is never present on the screen but is created by the viewer's own retina which is too slow to follow the individual light points. The eye can only respond to the rushing light points as meaningless flicker, watching the screen passively without moving; the eye muscles, like all the muscles of the body, are immobile while watching TV; the eye axes no longer cross and the dreamlike state ensues. Only a fragment of the sensory system is active (visual and auditory), and of this sensory bombardment, only a fragment can be coherently absorbed and processed. For most of the sensory input, the brain can form no meaningful associations and is merely stimulated in a mechanical fragmentary fashion. Since the brain is a plastically reflexive organ, it will develop into an instrument that reflects this kind of thinking activity. Yet while the brain falls passively into a trance-like state, TV engineering ensures that alertness is maintained by the technique of *saliency*, those frequent visual and auditory changes such as bright lights, quick movements and sudden noises that bypass natural neuro-sensory defences and capitalise on the brain's natural response to danger. Adrenaline and noradrenaline – respectively the flight and fight neurotransmitters – are greatly increased without any change in the body's activity. No wonder then that after viewing TV that is not necessarily violent, children are frequently restless, irritable and aggressive.

Other cognitive problems include: a reduced ability to form mental pictures, the imagination being stamped with ready made pictures and associations; thinking in rapid and predictable patterns; the child is less likely to read, preferring comics and picture books; a reduced ability to comprehend what has been read; reduced concentration; delayed speech development with primitive vocabulary and superficial and stereotypical answers to simple questions; short- and long-term damage to learning achievements. A 26-year study following children from birth through adulthood concluded that long term damage resulted from 1–2 hours daily viewing.[15] These vulnerabilities can affect a child's problem-solving skills and self-esteem in the classroom situation and could therefore indirectly predispose them to addictions in general.

Metabolic motor system, activity and behaviour

While watching TV, the muscular system is relatively immobile and even the eye muscles, which normally are constantly relaxing and contracting in accordance with constantly changing visual perspectives, are inactive. This inactivity replaces interactive and dynamic engagement with the outside world such as play, outdoor exercise and social time with friends and family. An inactive metabolism combined with snacking on high calorie fast foods has led to a huge surge in the prevalence of overweight and obese children as well as juvenile diabetes.[16-20] The gratification provided by passive entertainment requires no effort at all and when it becomes habitual, it weakens the child's motivation and desire to do things that spring out of his own volition. This results in a weakening of the child's will forces leading to low endurance, tolerance and resilience, making them easy prey for other addictions. A common phrase coming especially from children who watch a lot of TV is: 'I'm bored', which indirectly is saying, 'I cannot interest myself in anything, and I haven't the will to do anything'. In addition to boredom, TV may influence behaviour patterns such as aggression, restlessness, anxiety, fatigue as well as comic mimicry of TV characters.

John began to copy the gestures and mimic the speech of Sponge Bob Square Pants.

The effects of violence, language, sexuality and commercialism on the behaviour of children are well documented.[21-23] TV is able to penetrate the intimate world of the psyche because it is able to meet the insatiable need for novelty, excitement, comfort and pleasure of the soul for instant emotional gratification. Habituation to instant gratification, is a feature of the addictive mind, and could be expected to strongly predispose children to addictions in general.

There have been thousands of studies since the 1950s that have examined the link between exposure to media violence and violent behaviour, and the overwhelming majority has found a positive association. An average American child will see two hundred thousand violent acts and sixteen thousand murders on TV by age eighteen; programmes designed for children more often contain violence compared to adult TV; these acts of violence are frequently glamourised, accompanied by humour and depicted as a way of solving problems without consequences. Children

134

imitate the violence they see on TV. Preschool children cannot tell the difference between reality and fantasy, making them more vulnerable to learning from and adopting as reality the violence they see on TV.[24]

Rhythmic system and feeling life

Due to the close correspondence between the cardiovascular/respiratory systems and the life of feeling, the heart, circulation and lungs will be influenced by the effects of saliency on the autonomic system. Some studies have strongly linked the potential for heart disease to TV viewing habits in childhood and teenage years.[25] TV-addicted children find it more difficult to differentiate the 'real world' from the habituated screen world of entertainment media. They may therefore tend towards more escapist ways of being and social awkwardness, predisposing them to addictions in general.

Their feeling life is often superficial and heartless. Repeated exposure to TV violence makes some children less sensitive toward victims of violence and the human suffering it causes. Other research has demonstrated that watching violent media can affect the willingness to help people in need.[26]

Helping youngsters dependent on entertainment media

How do we, as guardians of our children and youth, living in a modern world, help those who are vulnerable to or who have succumbed to the compelling power of the entertainment media?

To begin with one needs at least to be open to the possibility that the entertainment media may be potentially harmful to the health of our children. This is by no means common knowledge, for otherwise children would not be allowed to watch TV for two to three hours a day! This idea may become more plausible when one considers the following: firstly, it is well established that the healthy foundations for the child's physical, psychological and spiritual life are laid down in the first ten to twelve years; secondly, it is also well known that the child, by virtue of his innate sensitive nature, is vulnerable in these years to impressionable environmental effects; thirdly, there is a huge body of current research that suggests that TV may be causing harm to children. The statement by the authoritative American Academy of Paediatrics that children under the age of two years should not watch TV because it can negatively affect early brain development, lends powerful credence to such a possibility.

On the basis of these facts, one could make a strong case for preventing children, as far as possible from watching electronic screens. This, in most urban families, is practically impossible. However, with effort this can and should be done strictly for as long as possible, but at least for the first three years of life; thereafter TV should be strictly controlled by measures that can easily be applied where there is insight and good will.

There are many committed parents who choose not to have a TV or DVD in the home.

If one chooses to have electronic media, every effort should be made to place the equipment in a room that children do not frequently enter, or in a concealed cabinet.

Parents who do not believe that banning of TV before age three is necessary or are not able to enforce it after this time should:

- restrict it to the minimum;
- control what programmes are watched. Non-commercial programmes as far as possible should be selected. In Sweden a ban on TV advertising to children is currently being debated;
- watch the programme with your child in order to monitor content, explain and correct realities, point out manipulation and discuss issues and points of view according to the age and needs of the child. It could also be helpful to encourage a questioning, critical attitude to the content of programmes.
- engage with parents of neighbours and the parents of the child's friends to agree on similar rules.

Every effort should be made to provide healthy interactive activities for children. Children who do not grow up with TV are often more social, creative, nature-loving, better playmates with healthier constitutions.

In situations of entertainment dependency and addiction, the approach is fundamentally the same as that outlined previously for any addictive behaviour based on the fact that the underlying cause lies in real needs that have not been satisfied.

In accordance with our management approach described in previous chapters, the first step requires an understanding of the issue at hand – that is, the entertainment media, its effects on children and its addictive potential. In addition, one needs to know something about the dependency spectrum and the nature of addiction. One needs to remember that addiction is invariably the child's best solution to resolving his discomfort on his own, a discomfort that invariably arose through a primary need not being met (see box).

Unfulfilled primary need → pain → blocking of the need → ensuing discomfort → the finding and adopting of a substitute gratification → appeases the pain briefly → secondary need → dependency on substitute agency

It is imperative to check out where one stands emotionally with regard to the child who is viewing TV and in particular how one feels about the TV issue. For as has been stated repeatedly, it is not possible to see the child's issue objectively unless one has cleared one's own issues first. What is your own relationship to the entertainment media? Do you yourself watch a lot of TV? Do you have a dependency on TV? This may need to be addressed before you can address the same issue with your child. Do you spend quality time with your child? What is the nature of your relationship to the child who is dependent or addicted to TV?

Understanding the child's needs and sensitivities is the basis for effective management. The silent cry for help of the TV addict is invariably that 'life is so tedious and painful I have to escape into a world of fantasy, so please help me find something that interests me'. Time should be given to observing the child carefully in the way described above, taking into account his specific nature and the specific environment in which he is living. His phase of development is of crucial importance with regard to best understanding and managing the problem.

Assess when it takes place, the duration, frequency of viewing, the degree of dependency and the warning signs of overuse.

The details of managing the entertainment media-dependent child or adolescent will follow the same principles as outlined in previous chapters, with specific attention given to weaning the child off his dependency and creating new and healthy boundaries for future viewing.

At the time when his parents consulted with me, John was watching on average three hours of TV a day. Both parents were very focused on their careers and were able to devote little recreational time to their child. The first step was to convince the parents that the child had an addiction and that this was a direct result of something very basic that he was missing. It was extremely painful for them to realise that it was their lack of parental care that had pushed John to find the best substitute he knew to satisfy his needs and longing for fun with his parents. Once they had come to terms with this, a therapeutic plan could be created. It was not easy for them to wean the child off TV; to begin with his behaviour deteriorated, he became agitated, restless, bored and had difficulty sleeping; his appetite decreased and he lost weight. At the same time a healthier home routine was established; firmer boundaries regarding TV viewing were put in place and other activities that engaged his interest were provided. When both parents became more involved in the child's life, John was gradually able to forget about the powerful attraction of the TV screen.

A further step was to try and reconstruct the child's fantasy and imagination. This was done by outdoor activities in the garden and nature, through pets in the home, and through artistic activities, which the parents themselves started practising, such as pottery, clay modelling and painting. The child was also placed on a treatment with natural medicines and supplements to balance out neuro-hormonal overactivity and to harmonise metabolic functions. It took the best part of a year to rehabilitate the child, who was then able to integrate himself completely into his second year of junior school life.

In 1918, Rudolf Steiner made several predictions that if humanity fails to find the right ideas to further human evolution, several events would occur.[27] One of these was that if we fail to find truth in our lives, there will develop a massive mind control of humanity. We are witnessing today in the so-called free world the power of the worldwide media controlling human minds. It is not Orwell's dark prophecy of *1984*, where Big Brother controls individual freedom by overt oppressive power, but rather Aldous Huxley's *Brave New World* that has found fulfilment in today's world. Ours is a Brave New World where humanity chooses to be controlled by technology, entertainment and amusement, believing that this reality is more true for us than our own life reality.[28]

If we wish to protect our children from these mind-compelling forces, we shall need to find the right ideas to create environments for our children that meet their sense of innate truth and goodness.

Chapter 8. Computer Enslaved
Children and Young Adults

I gaze in awe at you, computer, an intelligence that opens up for me a world of immense power and freedom. Yet you are an intelligence and a power that is not mine, it belongs to someone or something else; when you shut down your power, I am shut out of your web of information and access. I observe the world shackled to and dependent on your resources and realise, I, too, am caught in this web of dependency. It is an intelligence that brings both freedom and dependency. I see our children growing up in your world of freedom and dependency and wonder what you are here to teach us. I wish to know who you are, computer, you who power all electronic devices that captivate our children. I wish to know how to tame you so that I can teach my child the true meaning of freedom.

—

There can be little doubt that electronic technology has opened the way to another form of soul addiction. Computer games, internet and mobile cellphone addiction disorders are not yet formally recognised as clinical psychological conditions, yet many clinics and rehab centres all over the world are treating them as full-on addictive disorders, recognising that the salient features fulfil all the criteria used to define an addictive behaviour disorder. For instance, computer users spend more time than intended online or playing a game, neglect other responsibilities, and create significant relationship discord because of their use; they make unsuccessful attempts to cut down the activity, and have excessive thoughts or anxiety when not computer engaged.

Daily experiences

Do you recall the irresistible pull to check your email or see who might have sent you an SMS on your cellphone? Do you remember looking at the latest glitzy cellphone with the latest features and feeling the urgent desire to have one? Have you been surfing the web and found it compulsively difficult to stop, thinking, I'll just go to one more site, and then ... just one more? Have you experienced the compelling hold of a computer game where you had to keep playing until you achieved your goal? If you can identify with any of these experiences, you will know from the inside the addictive power of computer technology. You will easily be able to appreciate how children and adolescents, who generally have far less ability than adults to resist the pressure of satisfying their gratifications, are so readily sucked into the controlling nature of electronic technology. Recall how a child on a computer game, the internet or cellphone, is so hooked into another reality, she just doesn't notice you are there.

Daniella is an eight- year-old hyperactive child who spends every day on her Sony playstation. Her parents allow her to play on the playstation because it keeps her occupied and seems to focus her.

A seventeen-year-old introverted youth who came to see me for a nervous tic and a hand tremor plays computer games twelve to thirteen hours at a stretch, with friends or on his own, holed up inside his bedroom; when the door is closed no one disturbs him. His computer world, he says, is his second life. He spends hours on the internet competing in multi-player games and has recently begun online poker gambling with real money stakes. There are places out of town where games are played nonstop for the whole weekend.

A twelve-year-old girl tells me that her first mobile phone was her 'ticket to life' and she would be 'completely lost without it'.

Although there are no exact statistics available, it is well known that more and more children and teenagers all over the world are spending increasing amounts of time playing computer games, surfing the internet, emailing and chatting on line with anonymous surfers. And increasingly the mobile cellphone is becoming the most intimate and commonly used object of teenagers and adolescents. A survey by the Kaiser Foundation found that American children aged two to eighteen years spend an average of 4 hours and 45 minutes daily outside of school plugged into electronic media, and 21% had personal computers. This amounts to two solid years of computer viewing in the first fourteen years of life![1,2]

Modern electronic enticements

Children and adolescents are exposed to a number of seductive electronic activities:

A *wide variety of computer games* are available: violent action, shooter, adventure, role playing, strategy, racing, sports, fighting, and puzzle. They all give the player two things: the freedom to release her imagination in a ready-made fantasy reality and the power to achieve, to compete, to win or to overcome. Although boys are more frequent users than girls, this is changing as programmes are designed to cater for the latter's needs: for instance, home creation, relationships, woman power, and so on. In recent years there has been an explosion in electronic media marketing directed at the very youngest children: videotapes and DVDs aimed at infants from one month old, computer games and special keyboard toppers for children as young as nine months old.[1,3]

The *internet* is a free and open worldwide information network all for the taking, potentially connecting every computerised person with any item of information as well as with every other computerised person on the planet. Young people are mainly drawn to the internet for its entertainment, sensation-seeking, commercial and pseudo-socialising value. They may be exposed to information and images that are totally inappropriate for their stage of development: for instance, violence, sexuality, propaganda of many kinds. They are actively sought out by manipulative and exploitative forces: commercialism, paedophilia and anti-social propagandistic agents. The internet also gives the user world freedom and world power.

Mobile cellphones are potentially the complete mobile all-in-one personal computer unit: online messaging, internet, games, camera, music and entertainment centre. With one's cellphone at one's side, loneliness evaporates, boredom is erased and entertainment is always available. There is enormous power, prestige, sociability and freedom invested in a mobile phone.

Audio-electronics/MP3 players/iPods: Music and song move the soul in deep ways, soothe pain and provide pleasure and comfort. The components of beat, rhythm and melody, as well as the words in songs, meet the sensitive needs of growing children and create powerful resonance that evokes the wish for repeated experience. The musician and his lyrics become the inspired hero that is fanatically adored. This can fill the empty places in the soul with regular soothing gratification that results in dependency and addiction. Music and song may also replace the uncomfortable feelings of loneliness, boredom, anxiety or insecurity that silence creates in many children.

Gameboys, digital books and iPads: 'Just one more, my score is almost the highest ever, just one more' – these are words so often heard when asking a child to turn off their game, resulting in anger, frustration, disappointment or disassociation. At bedtime, some children now ask if they should turn their book off. The feeling of turning a page has been replaced with wiping fingers over a cold piece of glass.

Virtual worlds and avatars: Second Life and other virtual worlds allow users to interact with each other through avatars. One can explore the virtual world by meeting other residents, socialise, participate in individual and group activities, and create and trade virtual property and services with one another. This allows one to safely build a life and a being that is hidden from the real world. It allows one to engage in one's own unique fantasies. Although it is restricted for children under sixteen, it is thought that many children and teens play in this cyberworld. There are multiple other related games where one can live in a virtual world of make-believe.

Social networks, messaging, chatrooms: A child can become lost in the mass of information, gossip and plausible bullying in these virtual parties. Misguided information can create paranoia, anxiety, discomfort and confusion. These 'social' environments challenge empathy, the development of emotional intelligence and the ability to be 'seen'. Virtual hugs are not felt and eyes unseen do not touch the soul.

Dependency and addiction

Addictive behaviour in children and adolescents, as we have seen repeatedly in previous chapters, is an attempt to satisfy deep unfulfilled needs that have never been properly addressed. To add to this there is an inability to resist the gratuitous comfort offered to them by electronics. The child is desperate to seek relief from the ongoing soul discomfort that the unaddressed need creates, and finds a substitute 'partner' that may take the form of a defence mechanism (avoidance, denial, submission), an abusive substance, or a compulsive behaviour. The nature of these 'substitutive partners' in the addictive partnership are all different, appealing to the specific needs of the needy child: the craving for food consumed alone is very different to the need for alcohol imbibed in the company of others; nicotine calms one down when inhaled; the illicit drugs all have their specific nature and unique effects. These specific needs may follow different pathways: there may be the need for *soothing-numbing-comforting* or for *excitement-sensation-novelty* or for *escapism-fantasy*.[4] Television provides a visual-auditory escape from reality.

In our modern age, computer technology has arrived as the new compelling partner on the block, constantly promising to offer ever more powerful and interesting gratification to the hungry unsatisfied soul of the child.

Who are you, computer?

To understand this new addiction of our time, we shall need to understand something about the nature of the computer.

I began to reflect on my personal relationship to my computer and realised that I had no understanding whatsoever of how it worked, even though I called it my *PC*, my *personal computer*. It really is a very close and personal part of our lives, like a personal assistant (PA) or personal trainer (PT). I make great use of it to run my practice and dispensary, to store a huge amount of old and new information, to carry out my research through the worldwide web, collate information and word process the chapters of this book. Yet I knew nothing about how my thoughts and ideas were being stored by the computer's intelligence and then translated again into a language that I could understand. I realised that 99.9% of the population of computer users have no idea how computers work. Of course technology does not require us to understand how it works in order to make use of its functionality. I can still drive my car although I know very little about how it works. Yet knowing how it works allows me to feel more in control of the motor car; when something goes wrong, I may know where to look for the problem. It became critical for me to understand the basic principles of how electronic gadgetry works, not only to understand the growing phenomenon of electronic dependencies in children and youth but also to gain some command over this cultural force in our time that threatens to control our lives.

Electronics, electricity, world wide web

Computer technology is essentially based on *electronics*, a branch of physics and technology concerned with the behaviour and movement of *electrons* in a vacuum, gas, semiconductor etc. These electrons are the negatively charged particles of matter that under the right circumstances jump freely from one atom to another, creating a movement of electrons that we call *electricity*, the force that together with *magnetism* powers our civilisation.

Electricity is generated in power stations by transforming heat energy into electrical energy. Firstly, stored sun energy in the form of coal, gas or oil is released by combustion and converted to rotational energy by steam turbines. This energy is passed through huge magnets and coils and then transferred to electrons that are drawn out of the earth, thereby transforming it into electrical energy. All the power generating stations feed the generated electricity into a vast national grid that then distributes electricity to every industry and household in the land. Imagine this global spider web-like network that at its outlet points powers the millions of 'electronic devices of almost incomprehensible complexity entering every facet of human physical existence'.[5] We tap into this electrical network every time we boot up our computers. In addition to this *power web*, there are two other kinds of 'spider's webs' that harness and control global information – a *communication web* consisting of the *wireless* network of *radio, television, internet, cellphones and satellite communication* that uses wave frequencies of different kinds to transmit information around the world – and an *information web* comprising the *wired* network of *telephone and internet* . These three worldwide webs make up what Peter King refers to as the *technosphere,* in contrast to the *biosphere* made up of the living kingdoms of nature.[6]

Duad-Triad

Electricity can be switched on and off by means of an *electric switch.* Switch on, there is light and power, switch off, there is darkness and no power. This reality of the techno age based on the *on and off principle,* determines every aspect of our lives and our civilisation. *The power and intelligence of computer technology lies in its ability to switch its power supply on and off for every command asked of it and every action it takes, making use of the binary mathematical value system of 0 and 1 as its language to carry out these two functions.* How does it do this? Infinitesimal tiny electrical switches called *transistors,* built into circuits in a silicon microchip, control and manipulate the flow of electricity. The mind boggles imagining how a modern processor – the brain in the computer that handles most computer operations – can contain several million micro-transistors, laser-etched into a small plastic box measuring 40 x 40 x 3 mm, and becoming ever smaller with more refined technology The computer assigns *1* to a closed transistor that allows electricity to flow = *switches on,* and *0* when it is open and no electricity flows = *switches off.* From these 1's and 0's that are called 'bits', a computer can create any number as long as it has enough transistors grouped together to hold all the 1's and 0's. It can likewise create any words by assigning a specific sequence of 1's and 0's to each alphabetic character. Thus all information, in the form of numbers, words, graphics, pictures and music is stored in and manipulated in the form of different combinations of these two digital binary numbers. These billions of electrical pulses passing every second through your PC, give us the impression that we are reading whole letters, numbers and images, whereas in reality it is only information in bits.[7] *Computer technology fundamentally rests on the mathematical binary system expressing itself through a micro-electrical system and storing information magnetically in hard drives.* All our modern day computer technology, personal computers, mobile cellphones, digital cameras, MP3 players and certainly more to come, are based on this world intelligence that operates through the duality of *positive-negative, on-off, light-darkness.*

It is important to realise that the intelligence that lies behind the reality of the *duad* is true only for the material world of which the world of technology is a part, not for the realm of living nature where the *triad* prevails. Polarity only exists in a mechanistic world of cause and effect. A switch is either on or off, nothing in between. In the human world there is never only black and white, there is always a third force of equilibrium and balance that regulates and prevents systems from slipping into either extreme. Thus the healthy heart contracts to a certain point, then there is a pause, then the heart expands to a certain point and so on; it is like that with all biological systems; the healthy soul may feel down for a while but before it reaches pathological depression something shifts and one feels up again. An invisible regulating principle, operative in all biological and psychological human systems, holds the balance between the too much and the too little.

In Chapter 3 we described a system of rhythmic activities in the human organism that balanced out and regulated two alternating and opposite systems: the rhythmic system is constantly harmonising the contractile, centripetal nature of the neuro-sensory system with the expansive and centrifugal nature of the metabolic-motor system. This rhythmic system we saw is also finely tuned to the feeling activities of the soul.

This homeostatic balancing principle is invested on the biological level in the rhythmic activities of the body, on the psychological level in the feeling life of the soul. On the mental-spiritual level, it is present in the *I* nature or *Self* of the human being, and when it is absent or less present, as happens in all addictive tendencies, the duality intelligence takes over, resulting in harmful polarities that were described in previous chapters. The Self abdicates its central position and allows the drug effects to dominate the human system.

Earthly-cosmic

We have described addictive behaviour as an attempt to satisfy a need of the soul either by entering the body more deeply – earthly gratification; or by freeing itself of the body – cosmic gratification. On the one hand, the psyche of the child may engage with the body and the earth more deeply, drawing the child more strongly into material based thinking, constrictive feelings and power seeking activities of the body. These psychological patterns will gradually lead to functional and structural changes in the system, resulting in hardening, constricting and cooling tendencies (sclerosis, neuroses, earthly, material); one may say that *the light of the soul moves into the darkness of the body,* that *the light switches off.* We have seen this tendency in anorexia, sanctioned drugs and the earthly illicit drugs (amphetamines, cocaine, methamphetamine). On the other hand, the psyche of the child may move away from the body, seeking sensation, excitement and freedom in escapist and imaginative tendencies. These activities express themselves physiologically in warm, soft and expansive tendencies (inflammation, psychoses, cosmic, spiritual). Here *the light moves away from the darkness, the light switches on;* this occurs as we have seen in obesity, the cosmic illicit drugs (heroin, marijuana, LSD) and the entertainment media.

What do you do to our children, computer?

Whereas the compelling nature of the entertainment world forces the viewer to switch off her creative human powers and passively but willingly submit to the gratification that the world of entertainment provides for her needy soul, the controlling power of computers enables the user to be actively involved with the digitalised material for her personal gratification either of *empowerment* or *freedom*. By feeling empowered through winning a game, overpowering her adversary, having access to so much information or being in control of her social life through a cellphone, she connects herself more with her body, just as someone using cocaine feels more empowered in her physical being. By feeling liberated through free access to the worldwide web, and to a fantasy world of infinite possibilities that has nothing to do with the earthly world reality in which the computer user lives, she frees herself from her physical nature, just as someone using marijuana liberates herself from her bodily nature. Computer technology thus does what the designer drugs like ecstacy do: one part of the soul connects powerfully with the body – neuro-sensory system, eyes and the *digits* of the hands – leading to a desire for action or company with an impersonal companion; the neuro-sensory system draws the world into the body (see Chapter 5, p. 92). Another part of the psyche separates from the body – metabolic system, blood, emotions, fantasy – leading to an expansion of consciousness and a desire for heightened sensory and feeling experience; the metabolic system drives the psyche into activity and creativity.

Children and youth who are addicted to computer technology spend several hours every day being shaped by an intelligence that operates out of the electrical duality of 'on and off' and the mathematical duality of '0 and 1'. This is an intelligence that brings the growing and developing child on the one side too strongly into her nervous system, visual system, fingers and wrists; on the other side, disconnects her from the rest of her body and projects her into a second fantasy life that exists alongside her normal life. This may leave the middle ground, the heart sphere, with its functions of feelings and compassion overpowered and unable to carry out its normal regulating and balancing functions. One may well ask what this does to the child's physical, psychological and spiritual wellbeing.

Warning: potential side effects

A great deal of documented research on the effects of computer technology on children characterises the physical and psycho-social phenomena resulting from the misuse or abuse of computer technology and can be understood in accordance with the above picture. Here it is not possible to give a detailed description of the effects of computer technology on growing children. It is only possible to characterise briefly the potential hazards that may result from the overuse of computer technology and the risks of a broad range of developmental setbacks which may jeopardise their health.[8,9]

Physical hazards

Musculoskeletal injuries

Children whose bones, tendons, nerves, muscles, joints and soft tissues are still growing are at risk of developing *repetitive stress injuries* as a result of repetitive hand and finger movements conducted over long periods. Health and safety experts in government and industry, as well as numerous research articles, point to the risks involved through awkward positions of neck and back as well as through highly repetitive movements of hands and fingers. They also point to the precautions that need to be taken to prevent such injuries.[10] Armstrong and Casement describe why healthy ergonomic design and frequent breaks are essential for all computer users, especially children:

> *The computer is a kind of straitjacket into which the body must adapt itself. The eyes stare at an unvarying focal length, drifting back and forth across the screen. Fingers move rapidly across the keyboard or are poised, waiting to strike. The head sits atop the spine balanced like a bowling ball. Built for motion, the human body does not respond well to sitting nearly immobile for hours at a time.*[11]

Zolani is a high school student who was introduced to computers in his first year of school. He had free use of a playstation as a young child and was playing computer games every day for several hours. He developed pain in his hands which became so severe that he was unable to write or type. Lifting a cup, dressing himself or opening doors became very difficult and eventually he was forced to rest his hands for several months while taking strong medication to treat the inflammation in his muscles and tendons. This was a very painful way to break his computer addiction.

Schools are generally either unaware or in denial about these risks and many educational institutions do not provide ergonomic conditions for students working on the computer. Studies indicate that laptops pose greater risks to children than desk top computers. This is because the keyboard and monitor are attached together so that it is not possible to create a healthy posture, since either the monitor is too low, causing neck strain, or the keyboard is too high resulting in strain to arms and hands.[12]

Recent surveys estimate that the average American child spends about one to three hours every day at a computer, putting many at potential risk of injury.[2] Researchers recommend that children spend no more than forty-five minutes in an hour on the computer and less than four hours a day, both at home and school.

Visual strain and shortsightedness

It is well known that computer use in adults results in eye strain, causing symptoms such as eye fatigue, pain and burning eyes, tearing, blurring of vision and headaches. The term *computer vision syndrome* has been given to these symptoms.[13] In children whose visual systems are not fully mature until about the eleventh or twelfth year, the risks of eye strain are probably even greater. The immature visual system experiences the static two-dimensional picture of the computer screen in a very different way to the living, natural three-dimensional world in which the young child engages in an active dynamic manner. Visual-spatial awareness begins with movement of the body, first with gross motor control such as crawling, then with specific hand movements which lead to fine tuning hand eye co-ordination. The eyes learn to follow the hands but also instruct the hands in refining and co-ordinating fine movements. The integrated experience of seeing, touching and moving in three dimensional space allows children to appreciate visual forms as real objects and then to form inner mental pictures of their real outer experience. Perceiving small immobile objects on a computer screen takes place with very little bodily movement; the eye muscles, once they have adjusted to the focal distance of the screen, become fixed in this position and blinking of the eyelids is diminished because the eye is open wider. It is very likely that prolonged viewing of a computer screen will interfere with the healthy development of the visual system. When additional factors are present, such as inadequate and artificial lighting, viewing too close to the screen or at an incorrect angle, the risk of putting the eyes under chronic strain are even greater.[14] The incidence of myopia (near-sightedness) in children are likely to increase as children use computers for long periods at home or at school.[15,16] This will impact on the child's life in many ways, restricting their choices and activities and even impacting on their growing personality; myopic individuals tend to be more self-absorbed and closed off to the bigger world.

Experts in this field suggest that eye strain can be minimised by precautionary measures:

- provide lighting without glare, ideally natural light.
- the monitor should be placed about 60 cm (24 inches) from the child and about 20 degrees below the eye line.
- children should have regular breaks every forty five minutes and never spend longer than 4 hours a day on a computer
- internet research should begin only after the child has learned to read properly, usually after about nine years of age when they are better equipped to scan or read long documents.

Sedentary lifestyle health conditions

The sedentary lifestyle ushered in by industrialisation and compounded by computer technology is having a serious effect on the health of children. Obesity, adult Type 2 diabetes, heart disease and other serious metabolic illnesses are increasing exponentially in ever younger age groups. The rate of obesity among children and adolescents in the United States has nearly tripled between the early 1980s and 2000. The most recent statistics show that about 40–50% of school age children are overweight and approximately 15–18% are obese.[17,18] Type 2 diabetes, a condition rare in children, previously occurring only later in life, is now rapidly occurring among children. These conditions place the child at higher risk in adulthood of developing serious chronic health conditions such as high blood pressure and heart disease.[19,20]

Lack of exercise and movement that the hours at the computer contribute, is regarded as a major factor in the rising incidence of these conditions. Many hours in front of TV and computers means less time actively playing and engaging in sporting activities. Exercise has long been known to advance health and improve learning. There is a great deal of evidence to suggest that exercise stimulates sensory and intellectual development and the lack of it places children at greater risk of developmental delays, learning difficulties and attention disorders.[21]

Possible side effects from toxic emissions and electromagnetic radiation

Computers contain many toxic chemicals such as lead, arsenic, cadmium, beryllium and mercury. As many as twenty-one chemicals are released by new computers and visual display terminals and take from one to two weeks to dissipate completely. In a closed indoor environment, children will be exposed to these toxic emissions.

In addition all computers emit low level electromagnetic fields. Although there is no convincing evidence that such exposure is a threat to health, many studies cannot claim that there is no danger and call for further research.[9]

Emotional and social hazards

There is a world of difference between the impersonal relationship we have with a computer and the personal connection we have with another human being. Compare for a moment the interaction you have had with some person, with surfing the internet or reading a document on your PC. In the first place a dynamic interplay between yourself and the person takes place, whereby a variety of sensory perceptions, shades of feelings, a range of thoughts, memories, mental pictures and different modes of expression come about. Two whole people are interacting with each other. The engagement with a computer on the other hand, is, by comparison, one-sided, mechanistic, static, impersonal and soulless. Because the computer has no mind of its own there is no living relationship and therefore no possibility of a dynamic engagement. The visual perception of static figures on a screen, given meaning by thinking, sporadic feelings which may occasionally be engendered and the wilful tapping of fingers on the keyboard, are the sum total of our experience.

We therefore don't need rocket science to convince us that the emotional and social development of a child will be influenced and probably harmed by spending hours everyday on computers. In contrast, human contact, parental interest, interactive activities and social interplay clearly enhance and enliven this development.

Children who spend many hours on computers nurture a partnership with a mechanistic programmed intelligence for a substantial part of their waking life, depriving themselves during this time with living and active life experience which over years is likely to have a serious effect on their emotional and social capabilities. The building of friendships, personal commitment and community building may be seriously impaired in some children.

Dean, a shy and introverted teenager, speaks about his PC as his best friend. He can't wait to leave the supper table and to disappear for the rest of the evening into his room. His parents and teachers noticed increasingly his moodiness, withdrawal and isolation from other children.

The emphasis in education today is moving away from teacher-centred education to that of a computer-centred one. The computer has become the wise oracle, the teacher merely the 'guide on the side'. A great deal of the teacher's time is spent on computer training and computer programmes, and less time and space is given to the dynamic healthy interaction between teacher, student and subject matter. It is in such an environment – where the enthusiasm, individualised attention and innovative and imaginative input of the teacher is present – that the child can be inspired to learn, with often far reaching affects for her future life. Once again the mechanistic computer-centred intelligence operates within the framework of the duad, whereas the living human approach always works within that of the triad: the teacher, the scholar and the learning material.

The claim is often made that computers are highly motivating for learning. A close look at this issue shows that this usually requires the learning content to be embedded in sophisticated technology, where the sensory stimulation and entertainment value are the actual motivating factors and the educational subject is pushed into the background. It is not clear whether the supposed motivation enhances learning and self-discipline, whether there is an individual or gender motivational difference, or whether other educational methods would work better. There is also little objective evidence to show that computer generated motivation is long lasting, and more evidence that children become bored or jaded when the novelty of the programme wears off.

Numerous studies indicate that computers enhance social isolation and limit community building. The time spent on the computer removes children from personal encounters with parents, teachers and friends.[22,23] They are deprived of those direct emotional experiences which are regarded developmentally as the most significant maturing experiences of a child's life.

The situation changes completely when children work or play together on their computers. Here they engage with one another actively and interact emotionally using the computer simply to provide them with the content of their interaction as they together explore the internet, design projects or play games.

Intellectual hazards

Computers are designed to accelerate cognitive development and hardly connect with the child's emotional and physical development. In line with the child's natural developmental journey, learners in primary school should be actively engaging their feeling-emotional experiences as well as using their bodies, extremities and sense organs in the learning process. Computers usually provide far more information than the learner, at a particular age, is able to absorb, leading to an overload and even repression of her intellectual capacities.

Compare your own experience of planting a seed and watching it grow into a flowering plant with that experience gained by learning about plants from a computer. The latter makes use of controlled and contrived versions of reality, clever animation and simulated programmes that usually simplify and glorify mechanistically what is invariably a more complex and less predictable reality. In contrast, impressions drawn from nature or one's own imagination are always alive, personal and original, and always growing. A child who exercises her healthy creative imagination and fantasy is naturally curious, creative and innovative in her thinking and builds fertile mind pictures which provide a solid foundation in later life for the mastery of more advanced thinking.

Speak to experienced teachers about the change they have experienced as learners have grown up with computers; you will invariably hear how much more difficult it is for them to think creatively and form their own original mental imagery. The computer and multimedia feed children constantly with ready made images which immobilise their own spontaneous and naturally playful imagination.

Learners are naturally influenced by sophisticated technical computer software that may devalue their own authentic creative representation of the learned material. In researching and writing up projects they may focus more on mastery of computer skills and slick presentations and derive less value from the content itself.

Professor Sloan of Columbia University asks: 'What is the effect of the flat two-dimensional visual and externally supplied image, and of the lifeless though florid colours of the viewing screen on the development of the young child's own inner capacity to bring to birth living, mobile images of his own?'[24]

Very little research exists on the potential risks of computers to suppress or stunt creativity, imagination and the sense of wonder. However, common sense and our own daily experience can readily inform us how differently we respond to the living world of nature as compared to the virtual reality we experience through a computer screen. The sense of wonder that a child experiences when she herself collects an egg laid by a hen or the reverence that arises when she sees a butterfly emerge out of the cocoon woven by a caterpillar, lays the foundation for a deep sense for wonder, truth and social responsibility in later life.

It is well established that literacy, the ability to read or write, is developed out of speaking. First we learn to speak, then we learn to read and write. Speech and language skills continue to develop and are consolidated and expanded in the elementary school years through interactive face to face conversation with peers and teachers. Restriction of social interaction through increasing use of TV and computers is likely to lead to impaired language and literacy, a phenomenon that most teachers know about.[25]

Dean was one of many computer active children whose language skills were delayed and who lacked the ability to express himself clearly in speech or writing; his ability to comprehend fully what he read was extremely weak and he found it difficult to formulate clear and logical thoughts.

Jane Healy notes that language and literacy develop an ability to speak to oneself, which promotes academic as well as personal development.

This 'self talk' will help a child herself get through many problems. It is part of the inner armoury, that together with hard work, perseverance and overcoming challenges, leads to personal mastery. On the other hand technology that provides instant gratification, that turns educational projects into entertaining games and offers easy short circuit solutions to problems, amounts to 'electronically sugar coated learning' that deprives the child of discovering the joy and pride of self-mastery and leads to habitually lazy minds.[26] It becomes all too easy to download text and images from the internet, assuming this is knowledge self-gained when in fact it amounts at best to borrowing, at worst to plagiarising someone else's research. Much of our learning is of necessity knowledge acquired from researchers in the field, but there is a world of difference when this learning is internalised and we give it our own meaning, or when it is simply copied or rote memorised.

Overuse of computers have also been linked with conditions such as attention deficit and hyperactivity disorders; the nervous systems of certain children seem to be over stimulated by the rapid-fire sensory stimulation of multi-media technology.[27]

Moral hazards

Children exposed to computers at a sensitive and vulnerable stage of their development, are at risk of absorbing countless impressions that may be entirely inappropriate and often harmful for their level of maturity. They may be drawn into a reality that lacks an ethical and moral context or be persuaded to adopt a particular moral attitude. For instance most computer games are designed to feed the desire to achieve, compete or overcome an obstacle or opponent. Children who have not yet developed their own independent thinking and who have free access to the worldwide web will be exposed to sensational news items, online violence, pornography, bigotry, commercial propaganda and other inappropriate material.

Our responsibility

What is our duty and responsibility to children who are born into and grow up in a world of high technology that offers great services and promises huge benefits, but that is likely to damage the health of many children who abuse the technology? Dependency to computer technology is as devastating to the individual and to society as any other addiction.

We need to realise that computers and electronic gadgetry ideally are designed to serve the adult world and to replace and enhance, to a high degree of perfection, the automaton-like functions of the brain. Here the mathematical intelligence of the computer can greatly serve humanity. For children there is certainly educational value if used creatively and appropriately, and a great deal of educational material is now derived from electronic technology. Outside of school life, however, children and youth for the most part make use of computers and electronic gadgetry mainly for entertainment and gratification value. There is little understanding today of the forces at work in computer technology and therefore no care is given to protecting children from this danger. We must recognise the compelling power of computer technology to covertly gain access to the human psyche, threatening to bind humanity in an illusory grip of power and freedom. For when the vigilant self is not watchful, human nature can so easily succumb to the many temptations, comforts and gratifications that computers and other electronic gadgetry so freely provide. And children and youth by virtue of their undeveloped *I*-nature are most vulnerable to manipulation and exploitation.

Helping youngsters dependent on electronic gadgetry

We need to have a clear strategy to deal with children and youth at all levels of the electronic dependency spectrum. Most children seem to pass through close encounters with computer technology as a passing juvenile phase, seemingly unscathed and without becoming dependent. Yet can we be sure of this? Unless we, as child guardians, exercise extreme vigilance around their use of computers, can we be sure that their thinking, feeling and behaviour is not harmed by an intelligence based on the coercive power of duality, of either-or, of black or white, on or off?

There is a growing world view that children should be introduced to computers as early as possible: USA sales for pre-school software is a huge industry and programmes for babies as young as six months are booming. There is currently a strong lobby in Britain for obligatory introduction of computers at nursery school level.

I am uncompromisingly clear that pre-school children, before the age of seven, should not be allowed to handle a computer. This is because of the misalignment that takes place between body and soul when a young child watches computers for long periods. Any such invasive intrusion into the growing process of young children must, in my view, have a weakening effect on the developing organs and growing soul. Computer or electronic equipment should best be kept in a room that small children do not enter frequently.

As the child enters school and meets new friends she will inevitably become exposed to computers and other electronic gadgetry. We cannot hide technology from children. It is part of their world and they must engage with it. They must learn to master it, rather than be controlled by it. The question is, when do we introduce it to children, and when are they able to work with it in a way that is life supportive and not damaging to health? Children will awaken to computer technology on an individual basis, often in accordance with the degree of their exposure or their natural curiosity. When this happens the child should be introduced to the computer under strict supervision, explaining in simple language the reason for having a computer. Parents need to decide for themselves how far they choose to expose their children to computer technology. To do justice to this important issue, parents need to be informed of the potential hazards, in exactly the same way as they would first read the package insert of a potentially harmful pharmaceutical drug before they gave it to their child to ingest.

One should try to avoid *games* and the *internet* as long as possible, and parents should be aware of the type of games being played and the sites visited. Plugging into the internet is like tuning into hundreds of thousands of unrestricted channels, only a tiny fraction of which is dedicated to educational programmes. The internet is not just about education, it is also about marketing. The danger of a teenager having his own computer or powerful computerised cellphone is that you as a parent will no longer be able to monitor and control computer usage. This freedom of use undoubtedly creates a greater possibility for computer dependency.

Mobile cellphones today are an indispensable part of a teenager's outfit. It is a development of computer technology that takes the computer ever more deeply into the intimate life of the human being and is therefore potentially more harmful than anything that has come before. Children have the world of the web in their palms, instant communication, and the power of instant photography. I know of highly embarrassing situations where students photograph their teacher's underwear by surreptitiously angling their mobile phone as a female teacher walks past their desk and then cyber-circulating it through the community.

Mobile phones should be delayed as long as possible, at least until the discretionary faculties of a child are somewhat in place. Children before the age of ten or eleven usually have little power to regulate their own self-gratification and therefore before puberty the use of cellphones should be well controlled by the child's guardians.

Where addiction to computer, games, internet or cellphone has been identified, the same approach as outlined in previous chapters can be followed, with certain modifications.

A background knowledge of the nature of addiction and the developmental road map is always helpful.

Assess your own relationship to your computer and other electronic gadgetry. How dependent are you on this technology? What percentage of its use is work related, entertainment, or social? How do you feel about your children using computers? What do you notice goes on inside you when you see your child using the computer for two or three hours at a stretch? If you wish to be of any help to your child, you will first need to deal with your inner reactivity and put it aside. There may well be anger, hurt or resentment coming from another place.

Determine the kind of relationship you have with the child who you think is dependent on electronic technology. Do you have good communication with her? Is your relationship open and trusting, or based on your need for authority and control? Do you understand something of what lives inside this child? What kind of temperament and character does she have?

Assess when the technology is used, for how long, how frequently and whether there are warning signs of overuse.

Applying the methods described above, we can gain ever deeper insight into the child's inner world of experience; we place her in a certain phase of development and within a specific environmental context and we observe her overall profile keenly and with empathy. We try to slip into her skin with conscious imitation and to discover her desperate need for electronic technology? We see that the computer provides gratification for the child's needy soul, which she cannot find elsewhere. It may be the need for socialising, information, belonging, excitement, power or escape needs which she cannot realise through her own efforts, but which can effortlessly be accessed through the computer. Once again some primary need is missing, leading to discomfort and the quest for relief (see box over page).

> Unfulfilled primary need → pain → blocking of the need → ensuing discomfort → the finding and adopting of a substitute gratification → appeases the pain briefly → secondary need → dependency on substitute agency

Understanding the child's deeper needs and vulnerable nature is the foundation stone for effective management. In the words of a sixteen-year-old boy: 'The computer is my best friend, I can always speak to it, it opens up the world for me, I am never lonely and never bored, it gives me all I need'. When we listen to these words with respect and empathy, the child will trust your open heart and the first real step towards creating a partnership to deal with the problem has been taken. Making use of other conditions and guidelines described in Chapter 3 for effective communication, a great deal can be achieved within the home or school situation.

The details of managing the internet, computer or cellphone dependent child or adolescent will follow the same principles as outlined above. It will require partnership, motivation, commitment, contracts, accountability and realistic time frames. In severe cases it will need more intense clinical management, including individually prescribed medication for withdrawal symptoms, therapies such as massage, art and movement and specific counselling.

Zolani came to see me for his repetitive stress injury caused by long hours of computer usage. He was forced to stop using the computer and for the first few weeks was disorientated and dysfunctional: he was restless, unable to concentrate, suffered insomnia, was moody and listless. He agreed to a counselling session because I showed genuine interest in his computer orientated world but also challenged him that he had become enslaved to his computer. He experienced himself becoming a slave, tied down compulsively to the PC; he also saw within himself the master that controlled him. He was shocked to see himself caught in this power struggle when he observed himself imaginatively from a distance. Once he had seen this and had woken up to the reality of his addiction, he was able to commit himself to finding the strength to stand up to the master. He also had to realise that he had become a slave out of a need to be important and empowered. He felt this power only when he was on the computer. His new found strength was the true power that was needed to overcome his need for importance and power. We made a clear contract that once his injuries had healed he would permit himself a limited amount of time to use the computer in a constructive manner. Parents and teachers were also called in to be part of the contract although Zolani was sure that he could manage his addiction himself. While he was convalescing, he started a course of art therapy and discovered to his surprise that he could paint beautifully and enjoyed it. Four weeks later, Zolani was able to use his computer again, but no longer with his previous obsession. He also preferred to spend some of his free time painting.

The world of electronic technology has become an indispensable and intimate part of our culture and our inner soul life. It is like a life partner that accompanies our life path and children born into it experience it as a natural part of their world. Computer technology is programmed by an intelligence that operates out of mechanistic dualism, that same polarity that determines all addictive tendencies. In its inherent nature lie two fundamental aspects of the human being: freedom and dependency. It is the human self working out of the reality of the triad that determines whether we are served or controlled by it. Children and adolescents do not yet possess the power of this discerning self to protect them from potentially dehumanising forces that may abuse their vulnerability, corrupt their innocence and draw needy children into servile dependency and addiction. It can only be the discerning power of their adult guardians and care givers that can protect them until they develop the means to do so themselves.

Chapter 9. Shades of Addiction to Violence in Childhood and Adolescence

I cannot believe that children are inherently violent. Yet I observe children carrying out the most gruesome and aggressive acts on themselves and on other children. Where does this behaviour come from? How can we understand it? I wish to explore the nature of violence, how it manifests in our culture and how we can work constructively and creatively with it.

—

Daily news items

Acts of violence committed by children and adolescents have become commonplace events in our lives. It is estimated that between 25% and 43% of the perpetrators of violent and sex crimes against children are children themselves – some as young as six years old.[1] In 2006, eighty-two children were charged in South African courts daily for raping or indecently assaulting other children. An increasing number of high school students in many countries now carry a knife, razor, firearm or other weapon on them on a regular basis and frequently bring these weapons to school. In South African schools many teachers are having to handle aggression and violence in the classroom as a part of daily school life, and school pupils stabbed to death by fellow pupils are frequently reported. While child-on-child violence is becoming endemic world-wide, self-inflicted violence directed among children is also increasing exponentially. Children are inflicting injuries on themselves by cutting and other means, and committing suicide at a steadily increasing rate. Suicidal behaviour is increasing in many countries, developed and developing alike. In Canada and Australia, suicide is second only to accidents as the most common cause of death in children and adolescents aged ten to nineteen, and in the USA it is the third most common cause of death in youth.[2,3]

In this chapter we will look at the different shades of violence in children, the nature of violence as a human and world phenomenon and attempt to understand why it is happening and what we can do about it.

Our own experience of violence

If we are willing to look within, we will probably find a place where some shade of violence and aggression is present. It may surface when we are irritated or frustrated about something, when we feel hurt or rejected or when we feel threatened by some potential danger. It rises up from some hidden place, usually so quickly we have no time to stop it, proceeding to attack whoever or whatever happens to be the target of the anger. It could be another person who pressed our buttons, the cat we tripped over when we were feeling down and out, or our own self that we blame or criticise for doing something wrong or not doing something right.

In our everyday life, we are exposed to many varied expressions of violent and aggressive behaviour. Human nature expresses its displeasure through various shades of anger. We may experience this in our home life, in our schools, on the road, in every kind of social situation wherever there is human interaction. The news and entertainment media provide us with a constant supply of violent stories and pictures that feed into the insatiable desire that many people have for sensationalistic violence. We may notice that some children have a striking interest for bloodthirsty stories and are easily drawn into dangerous exploits, whereas others shy away from anything violent.

We shall examine the different expressions of aggressive behaviour especially as they manifest in children and adolescents.

Pictures of violence

There are many forms and gradations of aggressive behaviour that children and adolescents manifest, ranging from healthy defiance in a choleric two year old, to compulsive violent psychopathic behaviour that can be classified as an addictive tendency to violence. The various phenomena will be described for clarity as separate categories but in reality they are often not so well demarcated and merge one into the other.

163

Natural unfolding of the will

During the first seven years, the growing child progressively asserts his will over his environment as a normal developmental process, establishing his own autonomy and identity and creating the standards and boundaries that are right for him. The screaming fits and tantrums of an infant can tyrannise a family and lead to serious breakdown in family unity. Children who are more choleric will often exhibit aggressive behaviour, pushing, pinching, hitting and grabbing toys from less assertive children. They have not yet mastered the will on the bodily level.[4] The 'terrible twos' are well known, normal expressions of oppositional behaviour that lead to growing independence. Children who frequently misbehave and then lie about their actions are afraid of the consequences. Young children who 'steal' things may still regard the world as their own playground and feel they are entitled to it all. Most of this behaviour is innocent and short lived, expressing itself later in strong willed children able to show initiative and creativity.[5]

The first seven years is the age of imitation, during which time the child establishes good or bad habits through copying the conduct of people he experiences in his environment.[6] Thus a child who is often spanked will quite naturally feel it is right to hit out at his peers.

In the second seven years of life, morality is established by learning to understand by example the difference between good and evil. A child who is habitually exposed to violent computer games where destruction and death are the overriding challenges, will frequently carry these lessons into his attitudes, feelings and behaviour.

The tenth year, as the border between a light-filled childhood and a fearful dark unknown outer world, brings with it a new experience of the self, whereby the child is confronted with the dark and light side of his soul. This period up to puberty is often characterised by expressions of aggression directed outwardly or inwardly (fighting, petty stealing) as the teenager grapples with huge moral tensions.

In the third period of seven years the adolescent must experience inwardly the conflict between good and evil if he is to master the healthy unfolding of his will. An adolescent who does not have the good fortune to be guided by a friendly authority may fall into periods of moodiness, hostility and substance overuse that fortunately usually end innocently and are regarded as 'passing phases'.

Reactive behaviour patterns

We all know about our own reactive responses. Watch yourself closely in the course of a day and you will probably catch yourself many times reacting automatically in a defensive or aggressive manner to some outer trigger: moodiness, irritation, frustration, anger, withdrawal, judging, guilt are but a few of the manifold reactive responses. How many times were they of an aggressive, critical or violent nature?

Reactions are reflex, compulsive and usually repetitive behaviour responses originating from survival instinct and earlier defensive coping mechanisms. On the bodily level any perceived threat results in a physiological defensive response (the fight or flight reaction) that assures survival of the species. The animal kingdom provides us with countless pictures of reactive behaviour patterns that display the relationship between a trigger and a reactive response: for instance a bull terrier in a fight with another dog will lock its jaws on the dog and unless you know how to pull him off he will not let go. The will forces in the form of instinct, drive and desire are reflexively activated in the reactive response. These are activities governed by the animal's psyche working powerfully through its bodily nature. Also part of the animal's soul life are all the sensory and feeling processes that perceive and experience pain or pleasure. The human being also has a soul body. In the reactive human being, this soul dimension takes over from the sober and reasoning *self* in an instant reflexive and unconscious action where it is invariably detrimental to human interaction. Whereas the *I* or *higher self* can direct us to refrain from eating when hungry or decide not to be angry when annoyed, the soul nature simply reacts in a reflex manner. Since the development of the *I* is still unawakened in children and adolescents, they continuously manifest reactive behaviour patterns in one of four ways:

- *Explosive reactions* are outer expressions via voice, gesture or bodily action that have an effect on the external environment. Typical outer aggression and violent behaviour fall into this category.
- *Implosive reactions* are inner repressed expressions exploding on the inside because of the fear of the cost of exploding outwardly. For instance, a child suppresses his anger habitually for fear of upsetting his mother. This has a much more damaging effect on his internal environment,

weakening organ systems such as the immune system and liver, leading to energy loss and fatigue conditions as well as a loss of self-esteem and self-expression. In these repressed reactions, the violence is directed inwards in a self-abusive manner taking a variety of different forms such as internalised anger or fear, self-criticism or self-hatred.

- *Secondary reactions* are indirect pathways for outer expression, created for the release of implosive reactions where the feelings are expressed obliquely as an underhand action to get at the trigger: sulking, lying, ridicule, gossip, sarcasm, cynicism, and so on.
- *Somatic reactions* seen mainly in young children are bodily responses that express the inner discomfort, for instance through tummy aches, rashes and allergic reactions.

At the root of all reactions, whenever they occur and wherever they originate, there lie *hurt feelings* and *blocked expression*. Understanding this provides a rational and compassionate way to deal with violence.[7]

Disruptive behaviour disorders

There are two main types:

Oppositional defiant disorder

This condition of defiance, disobedience and hostility typically manifests between seven years of age and adolescence although it may begin as early as three. Before puberty it is more prevalent in boys, after puberty the gender ratio is equal.

Brendan is an eight-year-old child of divorced parents who displays consistent negative defiant and hostile behaviour towards his mother and school teacher: He is an angry child. At home he is constantly doing things that he knows annoys his mother, refuses to comply with house rules, is touchy, resentful, oversensitive and frequently loses his temper; in class he is often argumentative, disobedient and disruptive, blames others for his shortcomings and struggles socially and academically.

This pattern of behaviour may occur temporarily in response to stressful situations and alongside other disorders such as attention-deficit/hyperactivity disorder. It may progress to *conduct disorder.*

Conduct disorder

This is a common condition in childhood and adolescence characterised by aggression and violating behaviour, and occurring at more frequently in boys than in girls.

6–16% of boys and 2–9% of girls under the age of eighteen years are estimated to show this disorder. These are often emotionally-deprived children where socio-economic factors, family dysfunction and parental personality and behaviour are significant contributing factors.[8]

Bulani is fifteen years old, lives in a low-income urban environment with a highly dysfunctional family. His father is alcohol-dependent and physically abusive towards family members. His mother works in the day and walks the streets at night. He has a long history of aggressive behaviour; as a younger child he displayed cruelty to animals, committed acts of vandalism and was often truant from school. He is morose, verbally abusive and displays unfeeling and callous behaviour to his family. He is aggressive and defiant towards his teachers; he bullies children weaker than himself, is often involved in fights with other children and on one occasion stabbed a fellow classmate. He is sexually active, regularly uses alcohol and tobacco and has started using illicit substances and hanging out with other anti-social youngsters.

The aggression may be expressed in various forms:

Animal cruelty

There are many shades of childhood cruelty towards living creatures: small children will chop an earthworm in two because they want to watch the separate halves squirming, pull the wings off flies and other insects or pull the cat's tail with obvious satisfaction. The vast majority of children lose their interest for sadistic behaviour at an early age and grow up without any obvious sign of psychopathology. Although it may occur as young as four years of age, serious and repeated animal cruelty is most common during adolescence and is seen more often in boys than in girls. It is often associated with neglect or abuse in the family and is carried out by children who have poor self-esteem, few friends, have bullying tendencies and a history of truancy, vandalism and other antisocial behaviour. Studies have found that many children, teenagers and adults who commit acts of violence and murder have a history of animal cruelty. Animal torture is one of the acknowledged common indicators in childhood of known serial and mass killers.

Bullying

This can take place in any situation: at home, in school, outside school and in cyberspace. About one in five school children are bullied regularly and around one in five bully regularly. Boys and girls bully equally and both can be targets. The bullying continuum as described by E.M. Field has a wide spectrum: from relatively mild bullying such as innocuous social banter, hurtful teasing, mean body language and mildly aggressive physical behaviour (pushing and shoving), to malicious gossip, social exclusion (personal or impersonal through electronic media) and harassment (sexual, racial, religious, and so on); then to more serious bullying, for instance, mobbing, extortion and bribery, damage to property, physical injury and violation through unarmed fighting, to using weapons of violence and ultimately murder.[9] Yet even the milder forms of bullying can be extremely traumatic: some children have committed suicide after exposing information or sexually revealing pictures of themselves were circulated in social networks such as cellphones, emails or Facebook.[10–12]

Field describes four types of bullying:

- *Teasing:* verbal violence is used in many different forms, for instance, name calling, insulting, harassing, threatening, phone and electronic abuse.
- *Social exclusion:* the target is excluded from individual or group social interaction, for instance, the bully manipulates the group to exclude the target from social activities.
- *Harassment:* repeated interference and intimidation aimed at upsetting and hurting the target through verbal, sexual or physical action.
- *Physical:* regular attacks of varied nature against the weaker person or his property ranging from indirect intimidation to direct aggressive action of varying degrees.

The bully can only exist if he has someone to bully. The bully needs a vulnerable target and a reaction that usually invites the attack. Similarly the one bullied can only be characterised as such if there is a bully that bullies him. Often a co-dependent relationship develops. From this one can see that the bully and the bullied are two sides of the same coin. The bully may become addicted to his behaviour because of the pleasure and gratification it affords him. The bullied is likewise dependent on his habitual defensive response, which is the attempt to protect what is vulnerable. Underneath the aggression, however, all bullies are unknowingly highly vulnerable individuals, who hide their vulnerability through outer bravado and aggression. This is usually the expression of a hidden bully that is constantly harassing and abusing the vulnerable side of their nature.

Delinquency and gangsterism

Children before puberty commonly have the need to form gangs and, empowered by the group consciousness, indulge in petty acts of vandalism like ringing on neighbours' doorbells, painting on walls and stealing fruit from the neighbour's garden. These are relatively normal and innocent developmental acts of expressing independence and emergence into the bigger world. It is only those children with more serious anti-social tendencies who will become gang members of violent street gangs. They usually join up through peer pressure and forming friendships with like-minded youth. Most of these are teenagers or adolescents who have a history of earlier poor school performance, behaviour problems and psycho-emotional instability. Invariably they have an unfulfilled need for a sense of belonging. There is usually some degree of family or social dysfunction, for instance, parental discipline may be excessively harsh or absent through lack of supervision and control.

Self-injury

This seems to be on the rise among adolescents and young adults and is three times more common in females than in males. It usually begins between fourteen and sixteen years of age but may persist well into adulthood. In American high schools and colleges, 12–14% of students have engaged at some point in time in self-injury and 40–60% of psychiatric hospitalised adolescents have actively engaged in such activity.[8,9,10] This does not include culturally-sanctioned behaviours like tattooing and body piercing, but intentional and repetitive behaviour aimed at harming one's body and resulting in physical injury. This self-mutilation is done through cutting, scratching, burning, pinching, skin picking, hair pulling or hurting oneself in some other way. This form of self-injury is classified as *impulsive self-injury* that tends to be psychologically motivated. It is a classic addictive behaviour that fulfils all the criteria for addictive disorders. Self-injurers are dependent on the self-injury in the same way as a heroin junky is hooked to heroin. It is the best way they know how to control their painful emotions. It may also be a means of self-expression: *I need your help./ Are you interested in me?/ Is your love really unconditional?/ I am in control./ This is who I am./ I hate myself and deserve to be hurt./ This is my way of punishing you.*

Major self-injury tends to be more dramatic and life threatening and usually occurs in psychotic or drug induced states of mind. Injuries such as self-castration and limb amputation are fortunately rare and isolated events.

Stereotypic self-injury refers to repetitive and self-stimulating behaviours such as *head banging, hair pulling* and *self-biting* and is associated with infant or childhood syndromes such as autism and mental retardation.

Compulsive self-injury is repetitive, habitual behaviour such as *nail biting, hair pulling* and *skin picking* that usually causes minor and superficial injury commonly seen in Tourette's syndrome and body dysmorphic disorder. Nail biting, hair twirling, cuticle picking or scab or blemish picking are non-injurious, compulsive habit-driven activities that usually does not interfere with normal life.

Cutting

This is the most common form of self-mutilation and therefore deserves special mention. It occurs in about 4% of hospitalised psychiatric patients. Most commonly fine cuts are made on the wrists, arms, thighs or legs with a razor blade, knife or broken glass. Less commonly the chest, abdomen and genitals are injured. Frequency may vary from several times a day to a single episode. Cutters give different reasons for injuring themselves: it relieves them from overwhelming negative emotions and tensions such as guilt, frustration, anger, anxiety, sadness, jealousy and loneliness; it is a way of momentarily reducing the internal pain and numbing themselves to the inner discomfort; they may be giving expression to the way they feel, namely self-hatred, guilt, self-punishment; or it allows them to feel something again when they have been feeling numb and empty. The cutter is either trying to free herself from her suffering by getting away from her body ('cutting is like being high or taking a pain killer') or she is trying to connect more strongly with her unfeeling body ('I need to feel something'/ 'I feel alive again'). There is a frequent association with substance abuse, sexual abuse, eating disorders, mood disorders and attempted suicide.[13–18]

Susan is an introverted fifteen year old whose mother controls many aspects of her life through her dominant character. She has high expectations for her daughter and ambitiously pushes her to achieve at the highest level as she herself does in her executive professional life. She always decided what was best for Susan, and was never able to hear what she was needing. She could not understand Susan's depressive nature and was always telling her to pick herself up.

One day a classmate told her that cutting the skin with a razor bleed could let out negative energies from the body. She tried it with trepidation and found that she did indeed feel better. Initially she believed she was actually getting rid of toxic substances from the blood, but soon discovered that it powerfully relieved her emotional tensions. She felt free of the constricting feeling inside and began a compulsive pattern of cutting herself whenever she felt particularly stressed.

Suicide

The suicide rate among adolescents has risen dramatically in many countries, increasing three to fourfold over the past thirty years. Suicide is the third leading cause of death in the USA for individuals aged between fifteen and twenty-four years of age and second among white males in this age group. Currently the rate is 13.6 per 100,000 boys and 3.6 per 100,000 girls. Below fourteen years, the rate is 1 per 100,000 whereas between fifteen to nineteen years the rate is 10 per 100,000. In children younger than fourteen years, suicide attempts are at least fifty times more common than successful suicides, whereas between fifteen and nineteen years the rate of attempts is about fifteen times more common than suicide completions.[2,3,18]

In stressful situations many children have suicidal thoughts and make suicidal threats. Most of these are innocent depressive outbursts and relatively few go on to attempt or complete suicide. Yet how can we tell which children are at risk? Previous suicide attempts, mood disorders together with substance abuse and a history of aggressive behaviour are high risk factors. Impulsive adolescents with conduct disorders are prone to suicide during conflict situations. Other high risk factors include despair, hopelessness and social withdrawal, poor problem solving skills, depression (especially in girls), perceived failure in high achievers and perfectionists, conflicts, arguments, fear of punishment, broken romances, rejection, humiliation, pregnancy, school difficulties, bereavement, separation compounded with substance abuse in psychiatrically disturbed and vulnerable adolescents. Highly publicised suicides as well as television programmes and movies depicting the suicide of teenagers have been found to increase adolescent suicides (the *Werther syndrome,* after the central character in Goethe's novel, *The Sorrows of Young Werther,* who kills himself). Adolescents who engage in self-injury are also at risk since 50–90% of individuals who self-injure also engage in suicidal behaviour.

Understanding violence

In seeking to understand the nature of violence, our personal experience of this phenomenon can lead us further to discovering the reality that lies behind all acts of violence.

Recall how you felt when you lost your temper, verbally abused someone or committed any other act of aggression. Almost always there is a trigger that provokes your response. It may feel as if there is something against which one has to defend oneself, something that was in one's way, irritating or threatening. It may feel as if it is coming from the outside or it may be arise internally from thoughts or feelings. A protector is called up to protect oneself against some inner or outer threat. But if there is a protector, there must be someone who needs protection. Most of the time one reacts so quickly, there is no time to think who one is protecting or why one is angry. While the protector may be visible on reflection, the one being protected is usually not. With appropriate training it is possible to recall the event and to consciously experience what happens inside just before the aggressive outburst. One invariably finds that prior to the reactive outburst there was an almost simultaneous experience of feeling hurt or feeling vulnerable. This may be deeply hidden, often completely unknown, yet it explains the reactive outburst as a reflexive and instinctive response to protecting one's vulnerable inner core from some imminent danger. Tripping over the cat evokes *first* inner discomfort, then irritation and finally the violent response; the mess on the table may feel as if the ordered person inside has been violated, calling forth an angry response; unfair criticism hurts the person inside who believes in fair justice and provokes an angry retaliation.

We thus see that *aggression or violence is invariably a protective response to hurt or the threat of being hurt*. Furthermore, it would appear that in all acts of violence or aggression there are three factors or agencies involved: a *threatening agent* – the cat, the mess, the criticism which provides the trigger, a *vulnerability* – he who feels hurt, anxious, intimidated, and an *aggressive protector*.

From this point of view we can survey the phenomena of violence as it presents itself on various levels of human existence:

Violence and aggression in nature

Nature provides us with many examples of violent and aggressive behaviour in response to threats of various kinds: bees are notoriously dangerous when their vulnerable hive, the queen and honey are being threatened; an aggressive dog will protect its vulnerable owner when it feels the latter is threatened; a predator will stalk its prey when the vulnerability of hunger makes itself felt. Survival of many species of plants and animals rely on the innate natural power and aggression of the stronger to subdue the weaker. In a balanced ecological system the law of natural survival ingeniously creates a self-regulating principle whereby the stronger will only destroy what it needs to survive, for if it were to completely destroy the weaker it would lose its means of survival. Thus after it has fed, the lion can walk peacefully alongside the antelope it will hunt when hungry. A sustainable partnership in nature exists between the strong and the weak, where violent and aggressive actions are a part of the natural cycle of existence. There are however also many examples of pure unlimited aggression that follow a different law; for instance, terriers will kill rodents reflexly and indiscriminately until they are all destroyed, to satisfy, it would seem, some kind of killing instinct.

Biological violence

There are biological systems in the human organism whose primary function is destruction and breakdown of potentially harmful substances or agencies in the service of the integrity and homeostasis of the organism. In order that the system survives, the violent and aggressive activity needs to be constantly in action. We see here again a protective response to potential danger.

There are three main systems that carry out this function:

- The *immune system* is a highly complex and efficient defence system present throughout the body comprising chemical, cellular and biological components whose function it is to destroy any threatening foreign elements. The lymphocytes are white blood cells whose task is to eliminate foreign organisms either by ingestion or by the production of protein substance called antibodies that, like missiles, attack and destroy viruses. Specific lymphocytes are known as *natural killer cells* on account of their superior destructive abilities.
- *The digestive system,* through its sophisticated system of chemical substances (acid, pancreatic and intestinal enzymes, bile secretion), liquidising muscular action and intestinal bacterial flora, is designed to actively and completely destroy foreign nature in the form of mineral, plant or animal food substances and to transform it into a form that can serve the human organism. These food substances are completely stripped of their physical and energetic qualities in order that the neutral substance can be reformed into nutrients that carry the human energetic signature. The stomach acid and digestive enzymes of the pancreas and intestinal tract and the bile of the gall bladder are highly destructive substances that violently destroy all biological foreign agents such as bacteria, viruses, fungi and other parasites. The bacterial flora co-operate in defence mechanisms. Mucous secretions lining the surfaces of all hollow organs trap bacteria and destroy them chemically.
- *Programmed cell destruction:* Every cell in the body is equipped with tiny storage granules called *lysosomes* that

contain powerful degradative substances. These may be secreted and utilised within the cell to regulate cellular metabolism, maintaining the fine balance between anabolism (cellular buildup) and catabolism (cellular breakdown). Senescent or damaged cells destined for destruction are eliminated in this intracellular way as well as by other mechanisms such as destruction within the spleen or shedding of old cells on surface linings.

These healthy homeostatic mechanisms may become disturbed by excesses or deficiencies of one kind or another leading to a variety of *pathological* phenomena. These are some of them:

- *Hyperacidity:* As a result of heightened stress levels and weakened mucus protection, the stomach produces excessive acid that may erode the lining, causing ulceration of the stomach. In some cases it may be violent enough to cause a perforation leading to death.
- *Inflammation:* This is a healthy defensive reaction of the tissues caused by some toxic provocation. For instance a thorn, a sting, bacteria or some poison will illicit a tissue response whereby defensive agents (chemical, immunological) in the fluid or blood system are mobilised to eliminate the biological violator. In the process however, the body's tissues can be severely damaged. Think of a boil that breaks down, causing severe pain and lack of function for days until healing occurs.
- *Auto-immune illnesses:* It may happen that the cause of the provocation comes not from outside, as in the above case of the boil caused by a thorn, but from the inside, from the tissues themselves. Something tells the defence system to turn on itself and attack its own tissues. For instance, in rheumatoid arthritis, the cartilage of the joint becomes the target of an attack causing serious disability. This appears to be the biological equivalent of the psychological entity of self-injury. This category of illnesses in our time is becoming increasingly more frequent among children.
- *Cancer:* This phenomenon expresses the opposite activity. Instead of hypervigilance leading to self-destruction, we

have the loss of self-care and self-surveillance whereby the immune system no longer recognises potential dangers and does nothing to remove injurious agents. Eventually the tissue cells are modified to the degree that they take on an autonomy of their own, growing wherever they wish and causing death and destruction in their wake.

Psychological violence

All the pictures of aggressive human behaviour outlined above can be looked at from this point of view. Aggressive reactive patterns can be regarded as a protective response to a threat or perceived threat to a vulnerable inner reality; for instance the choleric child has to overcome an obstacle that threatens to place him in an intolerable inferior position; a teenager grounded by his mother for some misdemeanour feels disrespected by the way he is treated and may become abusive and violent towards her; he may however also take out his frustrations on his little brother. According to the same pattern, some youth become bullies, others are cruel to animals, others become criminals and prey on vulnerable people, while others hurt themselves by some form of self-injury. However, here we see vulnerability on the outside, or the inside being attacked, rather than vulnerability on the inside being protected. How can we understand this?

The answer probably lies in the fact that hurt and aggression exist and belong together in the human psyche; they are two sides of the same psychological experience. When you press your thumb into the palm of your hand it creates an impression, if you press it too hard it will begin to hurt; the impression and the hurt are determined by the amount of pressure exerted. The pressure and the impression belong together, the one needs the other in order to exist: the pressure leads to some effect (impression or hurt); the effect must have its cause (the pressure). Thus when the grounded teenager feels hurt by the disrespect shown to him by his mother, he continues to feel hurt, perhaps long after the confrontation with her; he feels constantly as if something inside him is hurting him, disrespecting him. This can only be himself that is doing this. So how does he protect his vulnerable nature from this self-inflicted aggression? He becomes aggressive outwardly thereby diverting his aggression and projecting it towards an easy target.

The case history of Bulani illustrates this pattern: he suffered years of abuse at the hands of his father. This has created a place in his psyche that feels constantly hurt and abused by an abusive power within. This was copied from his father through imitative learned responses and became an active force in his own psyche long after the outer abuse came to an end. This phenomenon of *introjection* created in Bulani an aggression towards both strong and weak targets as his only way of taking the pressure off his vulnerable nature. He will continue to react in this manner throughout his life if he does not find a more conscious way of dealing with his vulnerability.

Another violent psycho-dynamic activity is the internal self-abuse that many carry out constantly on themselves when they criticise and judge themselves for doing things wrong or not doing things right. Even in its benign form to which most of us subject ourselves, the effect is undermining and pressurising, the cause is blaming and admonishing. In its more aggressive form and especially when it becomes habitual, this internal violent behaviour has a destructive effect on the personality. There is evidence to suggest that chronic internal violence of this kind results in the spectrum of auto-immune diseases that have been mentioned above.[19]

Survival of the fittest

From an evolutionary point of view, the strong survive by controlling the weak, who either submit or are destroyed. A partnership based on *power* and *control* is established, where a strong controlling partner subdues a weaker and more vulnerable partner. In order to survive, the weaker partner in turn will assert its power and search for a more vulnerable partner to control, and in this way the survival of the species is guaranteed. Partnerships in nature provide a sustainable balance of give and take; the mineral world gives to the plant world what it needs to survive which, in turn, provides the animal world what it needs for its survival. Within the animal world, partnerships based on the hierarchy of power and control, maintain an enduring natural order and balance.

We saw too that on the biological level, power and control is an intrinsic part of every homeostatic process.

Within the human being, the psyche is also subject to a hierarchy of power and control. Violence and aggression always exist together with subservience and victimhood: an abuser requires someone to abuse and a violent person needs a victim to take out his aggression.

Elements within the psyche can take hold of this natural law and subvert it to gratify selfish and egoistic needs with huge destructive potential. If desire for power and control become compelling needs of the psyche, aggression and vulnerability inevitably become dominant psychological dynamics, and these controlling partnerships will be created on every level of relationship: they play themselves out on the interpersonal, social, economic, political arena as history has shown us, as well as ecologically in our relationship to our planet and our solar system.

Our world is permeated with power controlled relationships that disturb the healthy and natural order of things: The entire spectrum of addictive behaviour is based, as we have seen, on a coercive partnership where one element of the psyche compulsively drives a more needy part to habitually gratify itself by means of some addictive agent or activity. Co-dependent interpersonal dynamics very often involve a dominant controlling partner and a subordinate submissive partner. The one who is hurt by criticism and does not like to stay in the hurt, reacts immediately with aggression; the vulnerable cat is kicked aside by the angry person who tripped over it; an aggressive self-critic chastises the one inside who has done wrong. Families, schools, institutions, communities and nations can be subjugated by a single powerful dominant individual or a group of controlling personalities. Apartheid in South Africa was a state-decreed collective oppression of one race over another. Our planet is being slowly destroyed by a materialistic mindset that would plunder nature's gifts for egoistic needs with little thought of giving back or preserving the healthy balance that nature's genius creates.

Higher command

Within the human being there is also the possibility of harnessing the natural law of power and control for the greater good of humanity. An understanding and appreciation of this law in nature will enable humanity to support the sustainability of the natural order on our planet. But this will require that the egoistic desire for self-enhancement and self-acquisition be subjected to a higher command that, through self-regulating control, brings about balance and harmony between all partners. This higher command operates on the one hand from a higher perspective, where the whole is seen as a sensitive, integrated balanced system, and on the other where the right care is given to attend to the needs of all partners in the system.

Such a perspective for instance will recognise what has been stated above, that in the human psyche, aggression or violence is invariably a protective reaction to hurt or vulnerability, projected either inwardly or outwardly. To prevent this reactive dynamic from taking control of the natural order, the right care of both the vulnerability and the aggression needs to take place.

Thus the introverted child who experiences inner hurt and violation is more likely to project it inwardly towards himself; acknowledgement and proper care of the hurt inner child will soothe the pain and reduce the self-injury. The extroverted child often projects this inner experience outwardly in this acts of violence towards others; understanding his frustration and taking appropriate action will help to limit the social upheaval.

It is this higher power within us that will guide us to a deeper understanding of violence and the proper way of managing it.

Where does violence originate?

With rare exceptions, I do not believe that children are born innately violent and aggressive. If this is true then where does this internal violator come from?

Constitutional and temperamental dispositions

Some children come into the world with strong wills and innate assertiveness. These children are called choleric children and exhibit strong individuality, and strong preferences. They often have so much power they feel hot and congested and can at times explode violently. On the other side of the scale, introverted children with less inner warmth and outer confidence feel discomfort most acutely and create the most powerful internal abusers.

Neurobiological factors

The body contains a number of chemical substances that communicate between the nervous, endocrine and immune systems as information carriers. These neuro-endocrine transmitters seem to be implicated in a range of psychopathological conditions. The bio-medical school of thought regards the body's chemistry as the originator of psychological processes. However, the psyche viewed as the human being's personal field of experience, having its own independent organisation and using the physical body as its vehicle or instrument, may be seen to have physical correlates in the form of chemical substances whose levels will change in accordance with emotional fluctuations. *Serotonin* is a major mood regulator. Some research has found lower levels in conditions linked with irritability, anger, increased impulsivity and aggression, especially self-aggression. Endogenous opiates or *endorphins* are the body's pleasure chemicals that maintain a feeling of wellbeing and reduce the level of pain. There is research that indicates that self-injurers have lower levels of circulating endorphins and that self-injury increases these levels to normal. This may explain chemically the addictive nature of self-injury whereby the pleasure opiate response caused by self-injury wears off leading to the need to repeat the act. This continuous overstimulation eventually leads to tolerance, habitual self-injury and ultimately addiction. The pain threshold appears to become higher so that the need can become more intense and more frequent. *Adrenalin* and *noradrenalin* are chemicals produced in response to stress, the so-called *fight or flight response.* Increased levels appear to be associated with impulsivity, aggression and self-injury. Hypersensitive and emotionally reactive individuals may therefore also show biological reactivity.[20]

Associated conditions

A number of other conditions such as attention deficit/hyperactivity disorder and central nervous system dysfunction or damage may be associated with aggressive behaviour.

Toxic environments 1

Inner dispositions will be reinforced and influenced by environments that are harsh and violent. As described above, the child in the first seven years will actively imitate and reflect in his behaviour what he experiences in his environment. In the following years, his morality will be strongly shaped by the examples of good and bad and by the morality of the authority figures he perceives around him.

Parental-home environment

Lack of parental care characterised either by negligent or absent parenting or harsh punitive parenting with physical, emotional and verbal abuse, is one of the major reinforcers of aggressive behaviour. There are many shades of neglect or abuse of children: any degree of chaotic, dysfunctional and violent home conditions, divorce, bereavement, substance abuse and psychopathology in the parents are risk factors.

> *Adam had loving parents but for the first two years of his life his mother was grieving the loss of her own mother, with the result that she was partly not there for him. His mother also believed that children should not be overindulged: it was short pants in winter and no sleeping-in on the weekends. He experienced this in therapy as harsh and neglectful and had to work at removing the harsh aggressor imprinted into his personality.*

School environment

There are schools and colleges that overtly or covertly foster violence, discrimination and intimidation. Bullying and favouritism is a tradition in many schools. Using canes and other forms of physical punishment, as well as intimidatory toughening-up initiation rituals are still actively practised in many countries across Africa, south-east Asia and the Middle East.[21] Other schools may have a written policy regarding bullying but in practice little is done to deal with it. Many schools employ teachers who have an intimidating effect on pupils. Without forms of checks and balances and resources for continued training and re-education, such experiences may have a devastating and lifelong effect on the soul of a sensitive child.

Ecological violence

The systematic worldwide violent plundering of natural resources must have an impact on the child's sensitive nature. What happens in the child's soul when he hears about or sees pictures of whales and dolphins being slaughtered for gourmet food consumption, of rhino horns being hacked off by poachers, of vast tracts of indigenous forests being cut down for timber causing mass destruction of insect, plant and animal ecosystems, or of oil-spill disasters in our oceans which destroy countless millions of fish and plant life?

Toxic pollution of many kinds are constantly being absorbed into the child's constitution.[22,23] Do the inhaled pollutants, heavy metal toxins, vaccinations, and chemicals in food, drink and medication – petrochemicals, pesticides, herbicides, hormonal substances and food additives – have an influence on a nascent aggressive personality? Could the poor quality of refined and junk food, the high levels of sugar substances, the sanctioned substances like coffee and alcohol as well as many illicit drug substances, all have the effect of intensifying violence in children and youth?[24]

Sociocultural factors

Children who grow up in urban and socio-economically deprived areas are more at risk of violent behaviour. Parental unemployment, broken families, lack of social support and community involvement are predisposing factors. The ease of access of drugs and alcohol may also aggravate the circumstances.

Toxic environments 2

We live in an epoch where aggression and repression are an intrinsic part of every society.[25] Economic imperialism through industry and technology dominate and control the lives of individuals and exert powerful influence on many nations. In the western world free commercial enterprise has led to an egoistic and aggressive striving for personal wealth and power that has created on the one hand, a powerful wealthy class that essentially controls the economic, socio-political, and even the spiritual life; on the other hand, a class of exploited and repressed consumers or want-to-be consumers. In many eastern and African countries, political state imperialism based on a repressive ideology or state control dominates and regulates the lives of individuals. In both cases, the evolutionary march towards individualism that began in the fourth century BC with the invention of writing has resulted in extreme one-sided development of individuality, that has led to a perverted egoistic striving for possessions and/or power. Our civilisation is ruled by a materialistic Darwinian hegemony where the human being is regarded as merely a higher animal that has to fight to survive. Aggression in the human being is seen, as it is in all creatures, as an inborn natural instinct that cannot be eliminated. It can be actively repressed through fascist actions or publicly condemned by branding the 'aggressor' an 'enemy of the state'. At best it can be diverted into less dangerous social activities such as sport, entertainment, competitions and awards. But it may run unchecked, leading either to aggressive impulses that manifest outwardly as crime and terrorism, or repressive tendencies that cause psychosomatic turmoil, resulting in illnesses of body and mind (organic illness, depression, addictions, and so on).

A society based on a view of the human being that sees the aggressive animal nature tamed and regulated by a truly human centre, will find resources to transform aggression into a force that can serve humanity.

Apart from the aforementioned sociological tendencies that have developed through industrial urbanisation, there are also a number of other culturally determined factors that implicitly or explicitly condone violence. These include: abortion, discrimination, media violence and dehumanisation through media training. These are issues of enormous importance in our time and cannot be left out of the topic of violence.

Abortion

Many societies have now legalised abortion. This is the sanctioned ending of life of a human foetus up until the twenty-eighth week of pregnancy. How does a child or adolescent regard this disposal of human life that they hear about or personally experience? Children carry an inner knowing of what for them is true and good that often cannot be reconciled with the outer world reality.[27] They do not yet have the rational and emotional capacity to deal with such issues, and conflicts of this kind may cause confusion and deep inner pain.

Discrimination

In response to perceived threats to their own safety and wellbeing, individuals, groups, associations and whole societies may engage in prejudicial attitudes and behaviour that lead to discrimination against other individuals, groups and sections of society. The individual, through no fault of his own, simply because he happens to be white or black, Muslim or Jewish, gay, communist, migrant, female or child, becomes a target of oppression that carries within it the seed of violence. Those of us who lived through the insidious institutionalised discrimination of apartheid, know well the violent nature of this form of discrimination.

Any kind of discrimination – and it lives in every society in one form or another – may become a potent fomenter of violence and hate. One may well ask what kind of anti-human forces are at work in these attitudes. Children caught up in these societal or cultural preconceptions and prejudices will easily be pulled into this partnership of violence, acting out according to their nature, either the role of the oppressor or the oppressed.

Media violence teaches children to be violent

As we have seen in Chapter 7, exposure to violence through the media begins as soon as children are exposed to television. By the time the average American child is eighteen years old, they will have witnessed two hundred thousand acts of violence and sixteen thousand murders! In the USA, children's television shows contain about twenty violent acts each hour. On average children watch three to four hours of TV daily. Eighty percent of children younger than age six watch TV, play video games or use the computer on average two hours daily. Two-thirds of Hollywood movies contain violence. Violent video and computer games may have even a more harmful effect on children since the player can actively participate in the violent action that is presented in a highly glamourised light. These games teach the player not only to kill but also to like it. Modern music lyrics are explicit regarding violence, especially against women, and even glorify acts of violence. Our youth are also exposed to violence on the internet where thousands of websites advocate violence, hate and bigotry. Current research has shown beyond a doubt that media violence is linked to aggressive behaviour and real-world youth violence.[27,29] The only people who dispute this are people in the entertainment industry. Studies have shown that media violence is one of the most potent factors associated with aggressive behaviour, more than poverty, race or parental behaviour. The majority of studies concur that extensive exposures to violence have certain psychological effects on the viewer. These are some of them:

- affects viewers of all ages, intellect, socio-economic levels and both genders;
- promotes a negative effect on human character and attitudes;
- encourages aggressive and violent forms of behaviour and leads to a greater likelihood of exhibiting aggressive

behaviour in later life. Children imitate the violence they observe through the media;

- influences moral and social values about violence in daily life; the child believes the world is a meaner place, overestimates the possibility of being a victim of violence and becomes more fearful;
- fosters the gradual acceptance of violence as a way to solve problems and bring rewards;
- leads to an identification with certain characters, the victims or the victimiser;
- perpetuates scapegoating of subgroups such as women as the subjects of violent and degrading pornography.

Dehumanisation through media training

In the past two decades we have seen in the USA a spate of horrific school massacres perpetrated by high school adolescents: in Pearl, Jonesboro; Springfield, Oregon; Columbine, Colorado, and many others. This is also taking place in other countries. Classroom murders are happening more and more frequently in every industrialised country.

It is a sociological fact that human beings have an innate aversion to killing their own kind. Research into battle warfare has proven that only few soldiers enjoy killing the enemy, and if their own safety is not threatened, most will fire to miss the target. The closer they come to their enemy, the more difficult it is to kill them. Because of this built-in aversion, soldiers have to be trained to kill. It is even less in the nature of the child to kill. Why then is child-perpetrated violence and killing on such an increase?

The compelling research of Lt Col David Grossman, a military psychologist, describes how the military methods and psychological effects of training army recruits to by-pass their natural resistance to killing fellow human beings, are at work in media and entertainment, in conditioning children to violate and kill others.[30] The training methods used are fourfold: *brutalisation* and *desensitisation, classical conditioning, operant conditioning* and *role modelling*. We shall briefly describe these methods:

185

Brutalisation and desensitisation

Physical, emotional and verbal abuse is used to brutalise and breakdown preexistent norms and values (intimidation, humiliation, hardships). Once the psyche has been desensitised of its natural aversions to violence and can no longer offer resistance, a new code of values and behaviour, that promotes violence, killing and destruction of the enemy is introduced. This becomes accepted as the normal and essential behaviour required to survive in the violent new world.

Through constant exposure to media violence, children from the age of eighteen months are brutalised and desensitised by the thousands of acts of violence of every kind that they witness. When you tell children about real life murders they are often completely blasé about it. Can young children really distinguish psychologically the difference between media violence and real life?

Classical conditioning

This is based on Pavlovian behaviour conditioning. Soldiers who are rewarded for their acts of violence learn to associate violence with pleasure. This was a common method of the Japanese army in World War 2, as well as the modern suicide bomber who is brainwashed to believe his martyrdom will earn him endless pleasure with heavenly virgins.

Children relaxing with their friends, enjoying soft drinks and pleasurable junk food while viewing vivid images of human suffering, violence and death, are also conditioned to associate violence with pleasure and reward. Many react to scenes of bloody and spatter violence with laughter and cheer as if they derive pleasure from it and carry on eating their popcorn.

Operant conditioning

This trains the recruit by repetitive stimulus-response activities to react automatically to a specific response; for instance, when they see a head bobbing up on the target range they instinctively shoot to hit it. They learn to react as quickly as possible to specific responses so that in the real life situation, this reflex instinct will kick in and protect them.

Every interactive point and shoot video game teaches the exact same conditioned stimulus-response skills, to kill an opponent. There are many examples of real life murders where a teenager reflexly shot an innocent bystander who happened to move or say something. And many children involved in these massacres were avid computer game players.

Role models

The drill sergeant becomes for the young recruit a kind of surrogate parent and protector who becomes a role model, personifying violence and aggression.

Violent movies often glorify a violent perpetrator, computer game players can identify with and act out violent role models, and youth murderers who are broadcast on TV become role models for copycat killers.

We see from the above that the internal violator is copied into the psyche of the child from different sides where, without the protective power of a higher command that has not yet developed, reflexive behaviour takes over. Any danger perceived, presses itself like a seal into the wax of the living bodily matrix calling forth the wide variety of uncontrolled, defensive or aggressive will-based reactive behaviour responses. In this unguarded space, the child is at the mercy of hostile forces that can enter and take over.

Addiction to violence

When aggressive and violent behaviour becomes repetitive, habitual and compulsive and brings relief to emotional discomfort, the addictive process swings into action. Violence becomes another means, a false substitute to address unfulfilled needs that cause inner pain and discomfort (see box). Thus animal cruelty, hostile defiant behaviour, bullying, constant fighting and the various kinds of self-injury can all be used addictively to try to relieve pain caused by an original need that was never addressed.

> Unfulfilled primary need → pain → blocking of the need → ensuing discomfort → the finding and adopting of a substitute gratification → appeases the pain briefly → secondary need → dependency on substitute agency

Brendan lives with his mother and hurts deeply that he only sees his father twice a year; he is angry at his mother for taking his father away from him. His aggressive behaviour relieves momentarily the hurt he feels inside and he continues to repeat this behaviour because he has found something that provides him with a certain level of gratification. If nothing is done to relieve his hurt, this behaviour pattern may become an habitual part of his personality and he will effectively become addicted to aggressive and disruptive behaviour.

Bulani feels constantly violated by the life style he has been exposed to from birth. His aggressive and violent behaviour gives him a sense of freedom from his abusive environment and the constricted feelings that he constantly experiences inside of him. His cruelty to animals and his bullying of other children help to relieve his inner congestion. He keeps doing these things because of the relief it gives him. Fighting also relieves his tension and he is drawn through this need to hanging out with gangsters who give him a sense of power and control over the weak and vulnerable, both those outside as well as his own vulnerability inside. This activity becomes embedded in his soul life because it provides an answer to the continuous inner hurt and discomfort that he feels within. He becomes addicted to this violent way of living as long as there is no other means of attending to his deep primary needs of being loved and cared for.

Susan feels oppressed by her mother's dominating nature and feels there is always something missing in her relationship with her mother. Cutting herself gives her huge release and seems to fill the void she has experienced for so many years. She knows she is harming herself, but it is more important for her to be able to breathe and feel without the inner constriction that she has lived with for so many years. She becomes locked into a cycle of habitual and repetitive gratification through cutting herself; she was only able to break this cycle when she discovered through therapy how to nurture and care for that part of herself who was missing the loving care of a mother.

We may notice that the offensive nature of violence is the one side of the picture; the other side is the protective nature that guards a vulnerable inner core and that will do what it takes to protect itself from danger. This may require that it becomes the aggressor when its safety is threatened. This inner guardian does not appear to be aware of the vulnerable person inside who continues to hurt from this hidden place.

We thus see that the child or adolescent addicted to violent behaviour is compulsively dependent on the violence to temporarily soothe the continuous feeling of hurt that lives inside him.

When we realise that *aggression and violence is invariably a protective reaction to hurt or vulnerability*, we can relate very differently to the situation. From this higher perspective we are in a position to understand why the child acted in this way and to deal constructively with the deeper cause of the aggression. This mechanism allows us to find the most appropriate and effective way of managing the violence.

Helping youngsters addicted to violence

There are many things we can do to prevent and manage violent behaviour in children and adolescents; it starts with acquiring an understanding of the situation in the broadest terms possible:

An understanding of child development and in particular the individual child's nature will go a long way to pre-empting aggressive behaviour in children. The choleric child who is rough and aggressive with a newborn baby needs firm, unyielding but loving holding, praising and encouraging his leadership and protective qualities; the melancholic child who retreats defeated by his new sibling rival requires loving kindness and warm interest, challenging him to be helpful and nurturing to the helpless new born infant. When one understands that the third year ('terrible twos'), the tenth year (the rubicon year) and pre-puberty are nodal points of heightened inner tension, one will feel more secure and confident in weathering these storms.[31] If one can create in the home and school a healthy moral environment outwardly and inwardly, one will be doing a great deal to offset potential aggressive behaviour in children and adolescents.

Assess your own relationship to violence. Through fine sensing and imitation, children will absorb violence and abuse into their soul and bodily nature. Is the child's aggressive behaviour telling us about the violence in our own souls? As parents and child care givers we need to check out through honest self-reflection how these two elements live in us. If we discover that we carry a violator in us, either externally (explosive violence) or internally (implosive violence), we should find ways to deal with it, for our future wellbeing as well as for that of our children. For there is probably no greater factor in promoting violence in children than the ongoing violent nature of parents. It will also be very difficult to understand the child properly if we carry judgment or other forms of aggression into our relationship with the child. We first need to acknowledge that this lives inside of us and make sure it is not interfering in any way with our connection to the child. Understanding the violence within ourselves is the best way to understanding violence in the child.

Be aware of early signs of aggressive behaviour and take pre-emptive measures. Repetitive behaviour patterns such as *violent outbursts, aggressive behaviour, animal cruelty and bullying* need to be confronted with care and understanding. When one understands that all these misbehaviours are reactive responses to hurt feelings and blocked expression, there will never be a place for punitive measures. One should try not to meet a reactive action with a reactive reaction. This will simply aggravate the soul experience for the child. The child needs to feel that you understand why he acted in this way. Just consequences appropriate to the misconduct then need to follow, which will usually be fully accepted once the child feels he has been heard.

Other warning signs such as lying, stealing, changes in physical or emotional wellbeing, unusual withdrawal, signs of injury, fall off in performance, depression, suicidal talk, and so on, invariably point to an internalised abusive psychodynamic pattern which needs to be addressed.

Assess when it takes place and how frequently, and no matter how severe it is, try to understand the needs and sensitivities of the child and realise that the behaviour response is a conscious or unconscious cry for help.

Through *conscious empathetic observation* and *identification* with the child – creating a physical-sensory-kinaesthetic, auditory-tonal, thought-ego profile in the manner described above – one can come to a deep knowing of the child's experience of himself and his world. This can be further enhanced by seeing the child in the totality of his environment and subject to the host of environmental factors listed above.

A clear understanding of the problem and the level of violence will determine further management. Most cases can be managed internally in the home or school environment, provided effective communication can be established with the child. This as always requires a partnership based on trust, which the child will only give you when he feels safe, respected and understood. The child-centred guiding principles described in

Chapter 3 offer an approach that underpins good communication with children and youth.[32] Books that deal specifically with these subjects can be used for orientation and guidance.[4,5,6]

Specific management of disruptive behaviour disorders, self-injury and *addictions to violence* will usually require professional assistance and sometimes clinical admission. The best outcomes will usually be achieved as described in other chapters through an holistic multi-disciplinary approach whereby the young client enters voluntarily into a contractual therapeutic programme held together by a team which may comprise a psychiatrist, psychologist, the health practitioner, parents or care givers, other therapists, teachers, social worker or other personnel. *Counselling* should always be an essential part of the therapeutic programme.

> *Brendan was referred to me by his schoolteacher who was finding his aggressive behaviour in class intolerable. When his mother brought him for our first counsellng session he was angry and abusive towards her. Much patience and tolerance was needed by both mother and myself to acknowledge his depth of pain that was living still unseen beneath his aggressive words and behaviour. He needed time and space to express his anger, draw and paint the violence he felt inside and feel completely supported in this process. Gradually he started to feel that we understood and respected his anger and allowed us to see the deeply hurt child hidden inside. Next he was helped in a simple way to see this sensitive child who was all alone, frightened and hiding so that no one could help him. He decided this child needed help and found another part that was willing to care for him like an older brother. Through acknowledging and opening up his vulnerability he slowly allowed himself to receive the loving care of his mother and teachers. His mother took more effort to do fun things with him and his parents resolved to end their animosity with each other. The aggressive behaviour as a reactive response to Brendan's deep hurt rapidly disappeared.*

The fundamental principles of managing the more serious problems of violence effectively rest on three pillars:

1. Understanding that behind the aggressive and violent behaviour there hides a hurt defensive child whose inner soul needs have not been addressed and who will need

outer support and inner skills to empower himself.

2. Changing the environment where possible from a negative, toxic and destructive one into a positive, healthy and supportive one.

3. Guiding the child to understand his issues and to acquire the inner skills and resources to help himself.

Children and youth are living in a violent world where we are seeing a grave escalation of child perpetrated violence. If we are to find ways of checking this rampant destructive force in our midst, we shall need to develop a deep and practical understanding of violence. An essential part of this understanding will require some awareness of the powerful anti-human forces that are a part of all violence. We shall attempt in the next chapter to explore the nature of these anti-human forces.

Chapter 10. Sexual Addictive Behaviour

I have a great respect for the primal power of sexuality. It carries within it the power to create a human being. It is a power that children should get to know in the right time and in the right way. Yet we see today how innocent children are exposed to distortions of sexuality, which awakens them prematurely and for which they are totally unprepared. I ask what effect this has on their emotional and spiritual development. I wish to understand the nature of sexuality and how it can be subverted to become deviant and addictive. I wish to explore those forces that exploit and manipulate sexuality in children. I wish to find ways to protect children from these forces that are anti-human in their nature.

~

The daily reality

I was horrified to discover some time ago that in South Africa eighty children are charged in courts across the country every day for raping or indecently assaulting other children. Police, prosecutors, social workers and child rights activists estimate that between 25% to 43% of the perpetrators of sex and violent crimes against children are children themselves – some as young as six years old.[1,2] Although these statistics are not scientifically validated in this country, this trend seems to be worldwide. In the USA, various researchers estimate the prevalence of rapes committed by juveniles at between 20–30% and other forms of sexual molestations at between 15–60%.[3-7] In Australia, one study reports that children are committing 40–90% of sexual offences against children.[8]

When I try to understand what brings a child to perpetrate these violent sexual crimes, I have to repeat that I find it difficult to accept that a child can do this out of her own nature. For violence and sexual desire does not come from the innate nature of a young child. In some way it must come from outside. Just as children will not kill out of their own nature, but can be trained to be soldiers by desensitisation and other dehumanising methods, so they can only perform sexual crimes when they copy, are trained or manipulated to do so.

A child can learn through imitation to do anything she perceives by virtue of the porous nature of her soul, whereby impressions and experiences are instantly imprinted into the resonating life processes where it is stored as memory and able to influence bodily functions.[9] From pre-puberty when the first unfolding of sexuality takes place, the window of the soul is wide open for sexual exploitation and manipulation. Children experience the awakening and maturing of their sexuality with the accompanying arousal, desire and need for gratification in very different ways. The more cosmic type of child who is less connected with her body and more connected with mental, artistic and spiritual pursuits, will be less awake to her unfolding sexuality. The more earthly child who is preoccupied with her body and the earthly life will be more conscious of her sexuality. For some children these experiences can be extremely intense and disturbing; they may feel overwhelmed by a part of their nature that they cannot control and can easily be influenced by outside agencies. They may express their uncontrolled sexual experiences in a more inward manner through *sexual fantasy, masturbation* and *pornography,* or more outwardly making use of some external agency that is needed to satisfy the sexual gratification, namely – *sexual exploration with others, exhibitionism, promiscuity, prostitution, bestialism, sexual abuse and rape.* Perversions of sexuality turn the objects of sex into objects for self-gratification.

All of these aberrant sexual behaviour patterns may take on an addictive character that carries on most of the time in a hidden and highly secretive manner. Parents are usually completely unaware of this desperate struggle going on in the souls of such children. We may find it disturbing to read about sexual aberrations in young people but in reality it is happening all around us and it is better, I believe, to be conscious of these phenomena than to pretend they do not exist.

Sexual activities that can become addictive

Masturbation

This is widely regarded today as a normal activity common to all stages of life from infancy to old age. However this viewpoint has not always been accepted. Freud believed that neurasthenia (an old term for anxiety, nervousness and fatigue) was caused by excessive masturbation and in the early 1900s masturbatory insanity was a common diagnosis in mental institutions. Even today it is commonly believed by many that masturbation is immoral and has a debilitating effect on the mind and body, an attitude that has led to destructive guilt and anxiety feelings of many young boys and girls who will carry these feelings into adulthood. No scientific evidence exists to support these claims, although an energetic weakening of the system that cannot be detected by conventional scientific measurements, cannot be excluded. Sexual self-stimulation is common in infancy with discovery of the genitalia and the pleasurable sensation that arises when these are touched. Later the child develops an interest in the genitalia of other children, parents and even animals. This curiosity may lead to episodes of exhibitionism, genital exploration and mutual masturbation. With the approach of puberty, sexual curiosity and masturbation often intensifies. It is one of the ways that children discover their own sexuality and satisfy their sexual needs before they are ready for a sexual relationship. Adolescents are usually forced by social restraints to control their sexual impulses; this produces powerful physiological sexual tensions that can be released through masturbation. Masturbation only becomes pathological when it becomes compulsive, when it is no longer under wilful control and when it hinders adolescent development or social interaction; in the words of a young client who could not control this urge: '*It is like something alien enters me and takes control of me.*'

Pornography

We may not wish to acknowledge it but our children are exposed to pornography and have ready access to it through the internet and on their cellphones. Normal sexual fantasy develops out of a variety of sensory impressions that are given a specific meaning and internalised as inner mental pictures with sexual associations. It is inevitable that powerful sensory experiences meeting the young child through the media of television, film, video and internet sites will make a deep impression on the malleable soul life of the child and create powerful sexual fantasies. This may become a compelling force to find ways to act out these fantasies. Pornography is the easiest and most accessible means today.

Today children can watch soft porn on late night TV shows and any number of hard porn sites on internet when their parents are not present. The internet provides teens with unlimited access to information on sex as well as a steady supply of people willing to talk about sex with them. Teens may feel safe because they can remain anonymous while looking for information on sex. Sexual predators know this and manipulate young people into online relationships and later, set up a time and place to meet. However, they don't need a sexual predator to introduce them to online pornography. It comes to them often unintentionally through porn spam on their email or by inadvertently clicking on a link to a porn site. Pornography may have a damaging effect on a developing child's sexuality by distorting healthy sexual relationships, dehumanising the individual as an object of sexual gratification and reducing the capacity for loving human relationships. It may, like soft drugs, be highly addictive for predisposed individuals, leading them to become desensitised to 'soft' porn and moving them on to dangerous images of bondage, rape, sadomasochism, torture, group sex and violence. The same client told me: *'I became totally hooked on porn and could hardly live without it'.*

There seems to be a direct association between pornography and sexual abuse, rape, and sexual violence.[10,11] Thus some children and adolescents who become addicted to pornography have a history of sexual abuse and some may become sexually violent.

Paraphilia

Sexual urges, fantasies or behaviours that are recurrent and sexually arousing may start before or during puberty, and may persist throughout life causing immense amount of self-humiliation, loss of self-esteem and despair as well as social and occupational dysfunction. Fifty percent of all paraphilias begin before age eighteen. Although these disorders occur predominantly in adulthood, their emergence around puberty challenge us as parents and child care givers to know something about them. There are a number of specific disorders:

- *Exhibitionism* is the recurrent urge to expose the genitals to an unsuspecting stranger, usually of the opposite sex that is invariably associated with sexual arousal and masturbation.
- *Fetishism* involves some non-living object (the *fetish* may be a shoe, stocking, panty, glove) that is the source of sexual

stimulation or is essential for satisfactory sexual response. The disorder usually begins in adolescence, although it may be established in childhood.

- *Transvestite fetishism* typically begins in childhood or early adolescence where the teenager begins to wear articles of clothing of the opposite sex in order to create the appearance and feeling of being a member of the opposite sex and leading to sexual arousal.
- *Paedophilia* involves recurrent intense sexual urges towards or arousal by pubescent or younger children. It occurs in adolescents from the age of sixteen years.
- *Sexual sadism* usually begins in adolescence and involves recurrent, intense sexually arousing fantasies, urges or behaviours in which suffering of the victim is sexually exciting to the individual.
- *Voyeurism* is the recurrent preoccupation with sexually arousing fantasies, urges and acts that involve observing unsuspecting people who are naked or engaging in sexual activity. This usually begins in childhood and is more common in males.
- *Frotteurism* refers to the rubbing of the pelvis or the genitals against a non-consenting person for sexual gratification. This is often done in circumstances where the victim cannot easily protect herself, such as in a crowded train. The majority of frotteurs are male and the majority of victims are female or children, although female on male, female on female, and male on male frotteurism exist.

In adolescents, these sexual aberrations may be a transient occurrence or may occur only during periods of stress or conflict, or they can become a deeply stressful addictive habit. Unless detected, the activity is powerfully concealed by the teenager as his deepest and darkest secret causing unimaginable self-flagellation and despair.

Promiscuity

Teenagers who have frequent and diverse sexual relationships are at risk of unwanted pregnancy, sexually transmitted diseases (HIV/AIDS, syphilis, gonorrhoea) and damage to self-esteem. According to the

American Academy of Pediatrics, more than one out of three American fourteen-year-olds have had sexual intercourse; among twelfth graders, 17–18 years, the figure is two out of three. Research indicates clearly that movies, television, music, magazines and in particular the internet are fuelling promiscuity in children aged 12–15. These are a few facts relating to exposure of teenagers to sexually explicit material.

- over 80% of the episodes of the top twenty shows among teen viewers contained some sexual content, including 20% with sexual intercourse;
- 42% of the songs on the top CDs contain sexual content – 19% included direct descriptions of sexual intercourse;
- on average, music videos contain ninety-three sexual situations per hour, including eleven 'hard core' scenes depicting behaviours such as intercourse and oral sex;
- girls who watched more than fourteen hours of rap music videos per week were more likely to have multiple sex partners and to be diagnosed with a sexually transmitted disease.[12,13]

Sexual promiscuity is always a symptom of other serious issues such as depression, anxiety, poor self-esteem, defiance, sexual and other forms of abuse. A teen who is out of control may use sex the same way as she uses alcohol. She may believe it will improve popularity and make her part of the 'in crowd'. If 'everyone else is doing it', she may ignore the consequences that can come with this behaviour. And in our time HIV/AIDS is the most deadly consequence of all, contracted most commonly by promiscuity and unprotected sex.

Adolescent cultural beliefs play a powerful role as to what constitutes normal sexual behaviour: many teenagers, especially boys believe that sex is not the ultimate expression of commitment but a casual normal social activity or that sex is a sign of maturity, social prowess and stature.

Prostitution

The sexual exploitation of children for remuneration in cash or in-kind, organised either by an intermediary such as a parent, family member, or other procurer, or initiated by the child her self out of a need for survival, is a worldwide problem. Globally, according to UNICEF, there are an estimated 2–10 million children both male and female, currently in prostitution. Worldwide, each year, another one million children are forced into the sex slave trade, about 60–70% of them becoming infected with HIV/AIDS.[14]

This problem confronts us daily (or nightly) when we drive through certain suburbs, in specific areas in towns and cities and even in rural areas. Child prostitution has different characters in different countries depending on social, historical, cultural and religious factors:

South East Asia, particularly Thailand and the Philippines, has become most renowned for the commercial sexual exploitation of children and child sex tourism. Trafficking in young girls is rife across the borders of Vietnam, Cambodia and China. It is also repeatedly claimed that Chinese men will pay to have penetrative sex with a virgin because this is believed to be a cure for AIDS. In some places sanction is given to prostitution by religious values, stressing the duty and sacrifice for children especially for girls; by supporting her family through prostitution a girl gains merit rather than bringing shame on herself and her family.

In South Asia, namely India, Nepal, Sri Lanka and, to a lesser extent, Bangladesh and Pakistan, there appear to be three main components: the girl child, religious prostitution and trafficking for sexual purposes. The concept of the girl child has arisen largely in India where girls have a lower status and limited opportunities for education. As a result they are more vulnerable to sexual violation, early marriage and unplanned teenage pregnancy. In various parts of India and Nepal, religious prostitution known as *devadasi* and trafficking in children is practised, while in Bangladesh, the rape of pre-pubertal girls hired as domestic servants is very prevalent. *Devadasi* cults derive customary sanction from oppressive upper-caste temple traditions. Pre-pubertal girls, aged between five and nine years, from poor, low-caste homes, are dedicated by an initiation rite to the deity in the local temple during full moon. After a girl is married to the deity by the *tali* rite, she is branded with a hot iron on both shoulders and breast. She is then employed by the temple priest. Sometimes, even before menarche, she is auctioned for her virginity; the deflowering ceremony known as *udilumbuvadu* becomes the privilege of the highest bidder. The market value of a girl falls after she attains puberty, when she is said to have no recourse other than prostitution. In Sri Lanka the emphasis seems to be around boys and sex tourism. Here the role of *Spartacus* guides provide male homosexual tourists with up to date information about the availability of sexual contacts in most countries; they were notorious in the 1980s, particularly in Sri Lanka and the Philippines, for giving locations where boy prostitutes could be encountered.

Western countries such as USA, Western Europe, Canada and Australia face the problem of 'runaway children' who are allured to find homes in brothels as young male prostitutes, often referred to as *rent boys,* or young female prostitutes. In the USA, the current prostitution problem continues to be seen as having its roots in the alternative culture movements of the late 1960s. It is claimed that many children ran away to join these communes but, on leaving them, found themselves unable to make any money other than through prostitution. Runaways from abusive situations and broken homes seem to be the major factors. In Britain, children who have been in state institutional care as well as those from dysfunctional and abusive families are more at risk.

Many factors have been cited as common precipitating factors in the lives of prostituted children: these include homelessness, housing instability, dysfunctional home life, substance abuse, educational and vocational failure, general psychological and emotional problems, poverty and intolerance of their sexual orientation. Their immaturity, insecurity and lack of the necessary street sense to survive alone, contribute to their need to engage in survival sex, in exchange for food, money, shelter, drugs, or protection.

In Africa child prostitutes are mainly the victims of social upheavals due to wars, conflicts, natural and man-made disasters, together with mounting impoverishment among African populations. In South Africa, HIV/AIDS which is decimating families, poverty and abandoned children appear to be major factors forcing young children into prostitution. In recent years South Africa has become an origin, transit, and destination country for children trafficked for the purpose of commercial sexual exploitation and forced labour. It is mainly North American and European citizens who travel overseas and pay to have sex with boys and girls, mainly 5–14-year-olds, that have been driving the multi-billion-dollar global child sex tourism industry.

In Latin America child prostitutes are mainly female abandoned street children. Every child prostitute describes horrific life stories – being forced into becoming prostitutes, raped by pimps, terrorised by gang members, becoming dependent on drugs of all kinds. They are all lost souls without a home and with no one to care for them, brutalised and desensitised by their vicious and degrading life situation. They face immediate and long term damage. Most immediate is the physical, mental, and emotional violence these children experience at the hands of pimps, madams, and customers including forced perversion and beatings. Long-term dangers include health problems, drug addictions, adverse psychological effects, and even death.

Juvenile prostitutes try to cope with their vulnerability in different ways: through anger and aggressive behaviour, through dissociation from their experiences, through delinquent or criminal activity where they want to be seen as offenders rather than victims, or through drug or alcohol abuse. More than three quarters of all child prostitutes abuse illicit substances – substance abuse in turn leads to higher risks of prostitution.[14]

Many of these children suffer from depression, post-traumatic shock and are twice as likely to have serious mental health problems or to be actively suicidal: 77% experience suicidal ideation, 33% harbour lethal plans and 14% have attempted suicide at least once. They are affected both by the trauma of their sexual activity, as well as by the distorted information their exploiters use to justify their sexual behaviour. Their feelings of shame, guilt and despair may lead to an escalation of their promiscuity or their engaging in other reckless behaviour.

Because these children crave love and affection they can be seduced and exploited by procurers who promise comfort, protection and understanding. Once the child becomes emotionally and financially dependent, she is introduced into a life of commercial sexual exploitation.

A common misconception is that a juvenile prostitute is a willing participant in her victimisation, when in most instances she is coerced by her life situation or seduced and manipulated into this way of life.

Sexual abuse and rape

In South Africa, the country with the highest incidence of rape and child rape in the world, between sixty to eighty children are raped every day.[15] And these are just the reported cases. In the UK, ten to fifteen children are raped daily. International statistics show that on average around 20% of all cases of child sexual abuse are perpetrated by children themselves. There are thus two sides to this serious social problem. The one concerns sexual abuse perpetrated by children. The other is the child as the victim of sexual abuse.

The phenomenon of child-on-child sexual abuse is recognised

as a widespread problem both locally and internationally, and social workers dealing with sexual abuse cases are observing an increase in this phenomenon. Child offenders, if left untreated, frequently develop into an adult offender. The literature indicates that an adult offender if left untreated is likely to offend approximately 380 victims in his lifetime.

These child perpetrators, who are always male, are not even old enough to engage in legally consensual sexual relations, yet their sexual behaviour can involve coercion, intimidation and trickery. Their victims are invariably younger, smaller and weaker girls.

There are a wide range of factors that may contribute to child perpetrated sexual abuse: children from all socio-economic circumstances appear to be at risk for sexual offensive behaviour, although many of these children live in overcrowded conditions. Weak family cohesion, dysfunctional family life, experience of abuse especially sexual abuse and poor parent child relationships, in particular father–son relationships, appear to be factors. Patriarchal attitudes could increase the likelihood of boys believing that they have a 'right' to abuse female children. Families that are not open about sexual matters, may lead children to explore sexuality in an inappropriate and abusive manner. Exposure to inappropriate sexual material in the form of pornography, explicit media exposure and the viewing of people engaged in sexual acts can lead to sexual experimentation and inappropriate sexual behaviour.

Children who are sexually abused will usually carry the mark of this atrocity throughout their lives. For they are violated by an act of intense egoistic human desire that is far removed from their nature. They are forced to engage in an activity that for them is innately untrue and perverse to their innermost being. They bear shame that they were party to this experience and live for many years under the oppressive shadow of guilt and self-blame. If they remember what happened they may feel loathing for themselves, if they have blocked it out, their bodies which carry the memory, and they will manifest the experience psychosomatically in many different forms.

Chissandra was troubled for many years by a host of symptoms for which she had consulted me over the years: recurrent abdominal pains, erratic bowel functions aggravated by stress, painful and heavy menstruation, sleep disturbances with nightmares and fluctuating mood change. When she was thirty years old she began her first serious relationship and started getting panic attacks at the first sign of intimacy. She wanted to find out if there was any hidden reasons for these anxiety attacks as well as for her continuous ill health. In her first counselling session she allowed herself to experience her bodily response to a typical situation that brought on her anxiety; she gave expression to this experience by curling up her body in a contracted foetal-like position. She then withdrew from this position and looked at the after image she had expressed physically a few seconds before. She looked for a long time, then broke down and sobbed uncontrollably; afterwards she was quiet for a long time and then told me what she had seen. She saw herself as a nine-year-old girl who had been sexually abused; she knew then that she had been raped by her stepfather periodically for some years. This memory picture was real and convincing, transporting her into the experience of the young child from whom she had completely cut herself off. A journey began over the next few months of learning to be with this child and listening to her anguish, as well as allowing herself to stay in the pain. Many painful issues had to be faced in her path to survival: reclaiming her child and helping her to integrate herself into the adult woman; the deep hurt of betrayal, rage and anger; how was she to relate to her stepfather now? – should she confront him? should she lay a charge? –; her mother must have known about it, how to deal with this realisation and how to manage her future relationship with her mother. One sister refuted the claims and believed she must be making it up; the other sister knew it was true because she too had been molested but refused to declare it.

Chissandra had entered a new reality, one that exposed on the one hand the evil intent of a violator, hell bent on satisfying his animal cravings, on the other, revealed the violated world of the innocent, unprotected child. Both were present as experiences layered into her subconscious memory body that she now had been able to re-member and call up to conscious awareness. And because this had now become conscious experience, the possibility existed that she could take active steps to protect her inner child from further abuse and to heal her from the trauma she had experienced for so many years.

Experiencing sexuality

Sexuality is not something most people readily speak openly about. It is usually regarded as a very personal and intimate matter that needs no sharing with other people. Many people feel ashamed or embarrassed to speak about it and therefore naturally uncomfortable speaking about such matters with their children. This is completely understandable if one is not comfortable with one's own sexuality and there are many reasons why people are reluctant to go there openly. The sexual impulse is of a very primal nature touching us somewhere at the core of our being, in a place where we are most vulnerable. The way in which children are exposed to sexuality in their home environment will have a powerful formative effect on the way they experience their own sexuality. A child who grows up in the first years of her life witnessing the unashamed nakedness of her mother and father and feeling at ease with sexual matters, will usually be comfortable with her own body and her sexuality. In contrast a child who experiences nakedness as something to hide and sexuality as something to avoid, and associated always with embarrassment and discomfort, will invariably carry repressed feelings and inhibitions.

When one considers that sexual abuse in one form or another occurs worldwide in one in three to four girls and in one in five boys, we can understand the shame, guilt and trauma that is often associated with sexuality, making it such a taboo subject. It may be true to say that there is no aspect of the psyche that is more repressed than that of sexuality.

How do you feel about your own sexuality? Is it easy for you to talk about sexual matters? Do you remember your first awakening of sexuality? What was the environment of sexuality in which you grew up? Were your parents comfortable with their bodies and with their own sexuality? How do you feel about aberrant sexual behaviour. And how would it affect you if a child you loved and cared for was compulsively involved in some sexual activity?

Understanding sexuality

Building on our personal experience, some facts about sexuality may help us to understand the spectrum of sexual deviancy prevalent in our time. Sexuality embraces all three aspects of the body soul spirit continuum:

At a *biological level*, sexuality encompasses two main elements: *sexual identity* and the *procreative drive*. Sexual identity is the expression and pattern of an individual's biological sexual characteristics: genes, chromosomes, hormones, reproductive organs, external genitalia and secondary sexual characteristics. These will determine a person's gender, whether male or female, or in some cases a mixture of both. It will also determine the marked differences between maleness and femaleness: male bodies are usually heavier and coarser and tend to act in a more physical and wilful way than female bodies that are softer and finer and act more receptively and submissively. The body will provide the physical and chemical foundation for all functional activities related to sexuality, for instance procreation, ejaculation, menstruation, and so on, as well as for psychological activities such as the intense pleasurable sensations experienced when fine nerve endings in erogenous zones are stimulated. Instincts and drives are active at this bodily level.

At a *psychological level* it has to do with all matters relating to an inner experience of sexuality. It relates to a conscious awareness of one's sex or gender. *Gender identity* is a person's sense of their own masculinity or femininity and their relationship to the maleness or femaleness of someone else. It also includes sexual activity, affection, intimacy and eroticism. The latter calls forth bodily sensation at its highest level and there is probably no greater bodily pleasure than the arousal of an erogenous area of the body. Sexuality at the psychological level opens up powerful inner experiences, providing pleasure as well as emotional pain, for deep hurt and grief can be awakened by sexual experiences.

Because males and females are so different physically and psychologically, one may well ask whether these gender differences influence sexual behaviour.

The gender of the child to be born is usually of great importance to parents who may carry subconsciously all kinds of attitudes towards gender. For instance a mother who grew up with a violent and abusive father may carry subliminal fear in giving birth and raising a male child. A father who grew up in the same kind of violent environment may perpetuate this violence on his male children. Although male and female children seem to be more alike than they are different, certain differences have been verified: boys are more aggressive than girls who tend to be more submissive; boys respond better to what they see in front of them, while girls are better at picking up things from non-verbal cues.

We also need to be aware that many *gender stereotypes* persist as a result of social and cultural attitudes. These preconceptions and expectations have a powerful influence on the way many parents rear their children and strongly impact on the child's perception of herself: for instance females are the good housekeepers, males are the practical, technical ones; girls are more emotional, talkative and dependent while boys are more logical and show higher achievement motivation. As a result of these attitudes, male infants tend to be handled more vigorously, female infants are cuddled more. Fathers statistically spend more time with infant sons and tend to be more aware of their adolescent son's concerns than of their daughter's anxiety. Boys are more likely to be disciplined physically, and so on. Thus a child's sex influences parental attitudes regarding tolerance, aggression, interest, and so on.

Gender identity and gender role develop from a wide range of factors including bio-physiological determinants (genetics, hormones), physical characteristics (physique, body shape, genitalia) and social learning experiences from parents, siblings, teachers, friends and cultural factors. There appears to be a sensitive period between eighteen months and three years for the development of gender roles. Small children imitate the toys and activities that are for girls or boys, they see the women cooking and doing housework and the men going to work and fixing things in the home. Gender reinforcement also plays an important role (parental chiding such as 'big boys like you don't cry' and the different kinds of dress and toys). A young boy will try to emulate his macho type father who will encourage his son to behave in a typically masculine manner. Outside of the home, the peer group, schoolteachers and religious influences will put pressure on the child to experience herself and behave according to a certain gender role. Boys who dress up as girls or play with dolls may be considered a little queer. Finally storybooks, magazines and the media, especially television, invariably portray gender in a stereotypic way: men are active, dominant, innovative and independent, while women are passive, nurturing and dependent. TV commercials usually use women to advertise household cleaning materials and men to advertise beer.

At the level of the psyche, the forces of desire, sensations and feelings will drive sexuality in the untamed way it is driven in the animal kingdom. Bernard Lievegoed describes sexuality as a given force of nature that we have in common with animals and which we have not yet made human.[16] It is only the restraining forces of the spiritual realm that can curtail sexuality once it has been aroused.

At the *spiritual level*, sexuality is transformed into something that transcends the psycho-physical domain.

What does sexuality become when we have fully humanised it? Does it become pure love? At this point in human evolution, love and sexuality are very far apart. Love is expansive, warming, wants to open up and give to another. Sexuality on the other hand embodies desire and need, closes the individual in on herself and wants to take something from the other to satisfy the desire. Once satisfied the individual frequently shuts off from the other, unless there is something else to keep the heart open.

Because sexuality can become a gateway for love and deep caring for another individual, it has relevance for the spiritual life. Sexuality provides the psycho-physical foundation for the search for one's opposite gender, in C.G. Jung's terminology, for the animus or anima, and this quest for wholeness and unity embrace sexuality as part of a spiritual experience. At this level sexuality transcends the body, opening the soul to a high peak of human experience, where as neither male nor female, one feels united with all things.

If sexuality is determined only by the bodily nature of the *will*, namely by instinct, drives and desire, then sexual activity will be self-centred and socially alienating, contrary to the act of loving.[17] If the *Self*, using the higher aspects of the *will* – motivation, wish, intention and resolution – can guide sexuality by means of affection, tenderness, intimacy and eroticism, it can open the soul to heightened human experience.

Development of sexuality

A child discovers sexuality in infancy when, in the course of exploring the world she discovers her genitals and may derive pleasure from playing with them. As we saw, gender identity and gender role are usually already present by the second or third year with the display of typical gender behaviour, for instance, identification and choice of toys. By school age, the healthy balanced child will have a stable identity as a boy or girl, which remains throughout life. In early childhood, there is no preference for same or opposite sex playmates, whereas in middle childhood, children will tend to prefer their own gender groups.

A conscious awareness of sexuality arises in the child's soul some time before puberty, one of the most dramatic events in human development, as the reproductive and sexual organs mature, body hair appears and the voice changes. The onset of menstruation is a special and dramatic milestone in a girl's life, initiating the first experience of sexuality and the questions surrounding reproduction. This usually takes place before boys take an interest in sex – although commonly many boys become sexually aware through their first erection and experience of ejaculation or seminal emission (wet dream) during pubescence. During this period sexuality is strongly influenced by the biological processes taking place through the maturation of the reproductive organs as seen by sexually symbolic dreams.[18]

Children frequently begin their sexual exploration through sexual games, where they undress and look at each other or play-kiss with each other. It is important how one deals with these innocent pastimes, since heavy-handed authoritarian responses may create self-repressive and devious reactions. Fortunately for most children, adults do not discover the majority of these exploratory games and generally children grow out of them once their curiosity has been satisfied. Then puberty takes over bringing with it other issues that push aside the earlier curiosity.

Puberty begins about two years earlier in girls than in boys and is occurring at an increasingly earlier age. Girls especially are developing at faster rates and reaching menarche at younger ages. This phenomenon known as the *secular trend,* has become more prominent over the past fifty years and has been attributed to overweight, hormones and other chemicals in food, poor diets, socio-economic status, excessive physical exercise, better medical services, improved sanitation and health status. This trend also appears to be related to the degree to which the child wakes up to the world surrounding her, becoming in Steiner's phrase *erdenreif* or 'earth ready'. Dreamier and less grounded children and those who have been less exposed to media technology, sexually explicit movies, videos, rock music and an adult world, tend to have a more delayed onset of puberty.

One can expect the psychological effects of premature sexual development on the self-esteem and identity formation of teenagers to be significant. This in turn can lead to deviant sexual behaviour.

As the pubescent child becomes aware of the other sex, she also discovers the harsh world reality surrounding her. It is if she has been thrown out of her protected childhood paradise and now faces a grey and intimidating world. She begins to search for her own place in a much larger world, and may often seek out an older person of the same sex for guidance and friendship. During this time, she will also tend to mix with same gender companions. Girls will fluctuate more in their feeling life, either desperately needing to share their feelings with best friends or able only to express themselves in the safe world of the diary. Gradually, biologically orientated sexuality will change into an erotic intimacy-based sexuality. If this new relationship to sexuality does not occur, loneliness and alienation from the opposite sex may result.

Diaries may take the place of an understanding true friend, and are a refuge and a solace for the secret world of teenagers. Girls usually start diaries between twelve and thirteen, boys a year later and this may continue into late adolescence. This is often the time for romantically idealising someone of the opposite sex from a distance, often causing deep suffering and depression.

The extensive physical development that takes place during puberty creates a powerful awareness of sexuality that begins to shape interpersonal relationships. This is also the time when the teenager will discover her *sexual orientation,* recognising her dominant sexual behaviour pattern and sexual preference for a person of the same or opposite sex or both. She will want to explore and gratify her sexual needs in a socially acceptable way so that it contributes to the development of her sexual identity.

Sexual determinants

There are a whole range of factors that will determine how the adolescent relates to sexuality:

- *Age:* older adolescents are generally more sexually active than younger adolescents.
- *Gender:* boys generally seem to be more sexually aggressive, become sexually active earlier than girls, masturbate more often, have more sexual partners and intercourse more frequently. This may be biologically or sociologically determined.
- *Family:* dysfunctional family life, marital infidelity, absence parents, and parental attitudes to sexuality (either too liberal, or too repressed) lead to earlier and greater sexual activity.
- *Socio-demographics:* urban adolescents, especially those exposed to media technology, are generally more sexually active than rural teenagers.
- *Socio-economic status:* sexual activity seems to be more prevalent in lower socio-economic groups (overcrowding, lack of supervision, prostitution).
- *Educational status:* poor academic performance, early school leavers, limited opportunity generally leads to greater sexual activity.

- *Culture:* Eurocentric traditions have fostered an attitude of control and suppression of adolescent sexuality which has created a great deal of guilt and repression regarding sexuality; in contrast sexual exploration is encouraged in many traditional African cultures.[17] Western European teenagers become sexually active earlier than American teenagers, who are active earlier than Arabic and Asiatic teenagers; black teenagers in Africa and USA are sexually active earlier than white peers. Since the early 1960s sexual permissiveness has been encouraged by the student liberation movement in the western world, riding on the success of effective contraception and medical advances in the treatment of sexually transmitted diseases. Each culture faces the challenge of channelling the sexual needs of adolescents in a healthy manner; physically it must strive to avoid illnesses (sexually transmissible illnesses, HIV/AIDS); psychologically it must seek to avoid excessive preoccupation with sex that would interfere with education and social responsibilities and lead to the variety of sexual aberrations that have been described above.
- *Personality factors:* Self-esteem, inner security and sociability especially in the face of *peer group pressure* will influence sexual behaviour.[19]

What changes normal sexuality into abnormal sexual behaviour?

The literature describes a number of theories to account for sexual deviancy:

There is the *bio-medical model* that holds that high levels of testosterone increases the susceptibility to develop deviant sexual behaviours. Castration appears to significantly reduce deviancy. Chromosomal abnormalities were at one time thought to be a risk factor for the development of paraphilias, but research has not yet proved a connection.

The *evolutionary theory* suggests that because the more sexually aggressive males mated more frequently, those genes kept evolving, creating a *sexually aggressive gene pool* out of which sexual deviancy may arise.

210

The *Freudian psychodynamic theory* proposes that the superego responsible for self-control is too weak and the id that determines sexual impulse is too powerful. In addition it claims that the mother-son relationship, which is qualitatively different in sexual offenders than in non-offenders, plays a significant role. The mothers of sex offenders often display a love-hate relationship with their sons or practise covert incest by making their sons into their spouses. Sexual abuse towards girls may be a means of getting back at the mother.

The *cognitive behaviour theory* suggests that irrational beliefs and cognitive distortions help to initiate sexual deviancy. A teenager who was sexually molested for many years as a child regards it as quite normal to abuse younger children.

The learning theory suggests that offenders learn sexual deviancy from their environment. They may learn the behaviour from watching someone else exhibit the deviant behaviour, or by being subject to it themselves. They may also be exposed to long-term sexual indoctrination through multi media. Studies indicate that between 30% to 80%of offenders have been sexually abused. There are many offenders, however, that report that they have never been sexually abused, nor witnessed sexual abuse in the past.

The biography of a child who displays abnormal sexual behaviour will usually reveal on the one hand that the child's constitution in some way predisposes her in this direction; on the other, that some disturbance in the child's environment occurs that alters her healthy relationship to her own sexuality. Some of the environmental factors have been mentioned above: repressive parental and societal sexual attitudes, learned behaviour through an abusive upbringing, exposure to abuse, exposure to abnormal sexual activities, pornography and other long-term media sexual indoctrination.

Research emerging from a clinic in Gauteng, South Africa seems to indicate that most child sex offenders had not been sexually abused themselves, although they may have witnessed sexual or physical abuse. What they appeared to have in common was the influence of the media on their behaviour. In most cases absent parents and 'unmet emotional needs have turned television and the computer into a surrogate care-giver' – with disastrous consequences.[2]

Sexual addiction

All the above-described sexual activities can become addictive behaviour patterns when the child or adolescent compulsively and habitually seeks out sexual experiences to satisfy physical or psychological needs. Although not yet officially recognised as a psychological disorder, sexual addiction certainly fits the model of other addictions whereby a physical and psychological dependence develops and the development of a withdrawal syndrome occurs when the activity is denied. The addict is unable to control her sexual impulse, and she is compulsively driven to repeat the sexual act that seems to gratify her need. Even the strong feelings of guilt and remorse that may follow the act are not sufficient to prevent recurrence. The need for the pleasure or the appeasement of the pain is just too great to resist. Invariably hidden beneath the pain there exists a primary need that has not been assuaged (see box).

Unfulfilled primary need → pain → blocking of the need → ensuing discomfort → the finding and adopting of a substitute gratification → appeases the pain briefly → secondary need → dependency on substitute agency

---

The sexual activity may interfere with the young person's life, she may become morbidly secretive, depressed, anxious, guilt-ridden, despairing and even suicidal. Common to them all is the invasive action of some outside agency that takes over the will of the addict and compels her to act in a particular way. What is this outside agency and can we gain sufficient understanding of this phenomenon to know how to manage it?

Antihuman forces

Marlin, an eighteen-year-old adolescent, experienced the reality of pornography as a driving force within his own soul life. The porn sites that he visited, activated and fed his desire for sexual gratification so that it became a force so powerful that it completely dominated his thoughts, feelings and actions and prevented him from leading a normal life.

The desire for sexual gratification, present in every soul after puberty, is normally held in healthy boundaries by other restraining forces of the soul and spirit. However, the freely available porn sites on the internet and sexually explicit material in the multimedia, provide feeding grounds for the forces of sexual desire that reside in the vulnerable and impressionable souls of young people. These may be seen as forces in the world, which obstruct the healthy development of human souls, intent only on achieving their explicit goal of sexual gratification.

What, one may ask, is the intention of setting up porn sites to exploit the desire of the human soul for sexual excitement and gratification? If the motivation is simply a commercial one, then it would appear that an egoistic desire for riches supersedes the safety and wellbeing of children; either it completely overlooks the vulnerability of children and adolescents or it has no concern about the harm it causes them. This is bad enough. If, however there is a conscious intention to stimulate the desire for sexual gratification in children and youth, then it is something more sinister; for then one is forced to conclude that this intention is itself based on self-seeking gratification; this must be regarded as widespread paedophilic abuse of children. Such an intention has to be seen as something intrinsically malevolent, for there is present here a wilful choice to damage one of the most precious aspects of human nature – the innocence and vulnerability of children.

Any person who has the unusual opportunity to observe someone engaged in some sexually abnormal activity, will be forcefully struck by the change the person undergoes while engaged in this activity. The psychophonetic counselling process often affords both the client and the counsellor an opportunity for witnessing such a personality change when a client re-enacts in a controlled and safe environment what happens in her psyche when she engages in some such activity. One will then see the client opening herself voluntarily to another part of herself that is normally hidden and which only surfaces when the right circumstances are present. A completely different personality appears to take over, changing the way the way the person looks, her posture, breathing, thoughts, feelings and behaviour. Marlin became a vulnerable and needy person. However, he also discovered within his own soul life a power that seduces him into pornography. From the outside, this looks like a completely foreign presence; from the inside it initially appears this way too. Many such individuals will say they experience as if something has taken over, as if something alien enters them: '*I feel possessed by something that controls me.*' The same is true for any addictive behaviour. It is as if the object of the intense desire – the sexual object, the pornography, the heroin, the alcohol – enters the soul life as a personality that completely takes over the person's will, overriding any other motivating force of caution or concern.

What is this reality that is so powerfully present in the soul experience of every addict and that becomes graphically visible in the counselling process? Where does it come from? Is it something that enters from the outside or is it the resonance within the Pandora's box of the human soul that emerges as a persona when it is stimulated in a particular way?

Wherever its origin may lie, this is a force that may be called anti-human, being completely self-serving, socially alienating and destructive. Other than the gratification of the person's animal-like desires, it has seemingly no value for the enhancement of the individual's life; nor has it any apparent value for the advance of humanity. It belongs to a host of forces that seem to stand in the way of the healthy progression of human evolution.

In Chapter 12 we shall explore in greater detail the ongoing battle that takes place consciously or unconsciously in the souls of every human being, a battle between forces that would limit human potential and those that would enhance and expand her being.

Helping youngsters with sexually addictive behaviour

From the above it should be clear that if we have growing children in our care, these problems are not far from our own doorstep and workplace. If we are to deal with this new pandemic in our time, we will need to have a basic understanding of these issues, compelling ways of preventing them and effective ways of managing sexually addictive behaviour in children and adolescents.

As described in Chapter 3, an understanding of needs, gratification, dependency and the psychodynamics of addiction can be a good starting point. An awareness of sexual deviancy and sexual addictive behaviour in children and youth will tune one into the reality in which children today are living.

It is essential, as always, to *assess your own relationship to sexuality.*

This is not an easy challenge for any parent, teacher or therapist, but needs to be done if we are to offer children a healthy relationship to their own sexuality. If one is uneasy or uncomfortable with sexuality, children will immediately sense it and either copy it or react to it, with repression or rebellion. Once one has a clearer understanding of one's own sexuality, one will be in a better position to empathise with the sexual issues with which the adolescent in your care is trying to deal. As mentioned earlier, one also needs to check one's own attitudes to sexual activities, deviancy and addictive behaviour.

Sexual issues need to be discussed openly with children and adolescents. This is a step of critical importance emphasised by all experts in the field. Naturally the way this is handled and received will be determined by your relationship to your own sexuality. Children who can openly hear and speak about sexual matters from someone they trust, will have less need to follow devious routes in the necessary exploration of their sexuality. It is only in the spirit of open communication around sexuality that the potential dangers can be pointed out. Yet however open, liberal and permissive one is, adolescents regard this area as their private domain that we as parents and carers should fully respect. It is a privilege if a child allows you into this intimate sharing space, for they will only seek out someone to speak about such matters whom they feel has earned their trust and respect.

Parents and guardians need to exercise some control over their adolescent children with regard to their social life and contacts. This will of course depend greatly on the maturity of the child and the level of trust one has with the child.

Insight into child development is a prerequisite. An understanding of normal child development and in particular the healthy development of sexuality in adolescents will create a platform on which the nature of the individual child in your care can be understood. One will then be ready and more aware to catch the subtle changes that tell one that all is not well in the life of the child. For the child will not tell you there is a problem until it becomes impossible for her to hide it.

A child or adolescent that one suspects or knows has a sexual behaviour issue needs to be handled with great sensitivity. One needs to have first cleared one's own emotional sensitivities with regard to the child and her sexual issues before one can see the child objectively. A profile of the child's nature can then be acquired through fine observation and empathetic exploration in the manner described in Chapter 2. This child will also need to be seen in the context of her whole environment. What is her relationship to her parents, siblings and extended family? What happens in her school environment, in her contacts with teachers and other learners? Outside of home and school, what does she do with her social time, where does she go and who are her friends and acquaintances and other contacts?

Be aware of early signs of any addictive tendencies, when it takes place, how frequently, and no matter how severe it is, try to understand the needs and sensitivities of the child and that the behaviour response is a conscious or unconscious cry for help. Warning signs such as changes in physical or emotional wellbeing, unusual withdrawal, fall off in performance, severe depression, staying out late at night, frequent partners, exhibitionist tendencies, finding sexual paraphernalia etc, will indicate that the youth is in some trouble. One should be more attentive to adolescents who are inclined to want their needs immediately gratified. Children should not have free access to internet sites, and constraints need to be created for television and media technology where explicit sexual material is available.

Every effort should be made to *communicate effectively* with the child in accordance with child-centred guiding principles.[20]

Specific management of sexual addictive behaviour will usually require professional assistance, for it will invariably surface only when the problem has reached a degree of intensity that makes it very difficult for the child to conceal. However parents and guardians may well be able to intervene and assist positively if they understand the three fundamental principles of managing these problems effectively:

1. Understanding that behind the aberrant sexual behaviour there hides a vulnerable and needy child whose inner soul needs have not been addressed and who will need outer support and inner skills to empower herself.
2. Changing the environment, where possible, from a negative, toxic and destructive one into a positive, healthy and supportive one.
3. Guiding the child to understand her issues and to acquire the inner skills and resources to help herself.

The best outcomes will usually be achieved as described above through an holistic multi-disciplinary approach whereby the young client enters voluntarily into a contractual therapeutic programme held together by the health practitioner, parents or guardians, therapists, teachers, social worker and other personnel.

Counselling is an essential part of the therapeutic programme. As stated, I have found *psychophonetic counselling* to be especially effective in dealing with addictive disorders, helping the child to achieve self-mastery over forces that are hellbent on annihilating him.

> *Marlin was addicted to pornography. His father had remarried and several years ago he had moved in with his step mother and her two children with whom he did not get on. He felt like a stranger in the family, worsened by the fact that his father seemed more interested in nurturing his new family than in supporting and maintaining the relationship with his son. He was lonely, morose and withdrawn and found comfort and short relief in his private fantasy world of pornography and the ensuing masturbation. Afterwards he suffered deep remorse and would wait in anguish, mixed with intense and eager anticipation, for the next urge to visit a porn site. He was completely unable to counter this urge, which became progressively more frequent and he found himself trapped in an obsessive and compulsive activity that he felt unable to control.*
>
> *In his first counselling session he became aware that he was addicted to pornography, that it had become his lifeline to comfort and short-term happiness and that this was a substitute for finding his happiness from within. His wish was to find the power to counter the addictive urge and to discover comfort inside himself.*
>
> *Marlin experienced through recall being drawn into the world of pornography. He was guided to sense how it felt in his body when the first urge overtook him and to express this in a gesture. The picture he created was of someone with outstretched hands being drawn to something he was yearning for. When he stepped out of this position and looked at the after image he had created, he could see himself longing for the porn and the comfort that it gave him.*

What is it that pulls at your heart so strongly, forcing you into an activity that you know is not healthy for you? Will you be willing to step into this pleasure-seeking role to gain insight into this reality?

⌣

Having experienced being the needy person longing for comfort, it is not difficult for Marlin to play the role of the one offering him comfort. He becomes a most beautiful and highly seductive woman who entices him into exposing himself in the most vulnerable part of his nature. He steps out of this position and sees for the first time a personification of pornography and how he has become entrapped by it. He is overcome with emotion.

Will you continue to expose your vulnerability to a seductress power that feeds on your neediness and drops you the moment she has satisfied your physical-emotional needs?

—

Marlin realises that he needs a more reliable and less seductive partner and describes imaginatively a warm maternal comforting character that could be always present in his lonely times. He inwardly invokes this character, becoming this persona who approaches the seductress and firmly informs her that her services are no longer required; this new maternal character commits herself to taking over the task of helping and supporting Marlin in his vulnerable nature. She then turns to him, meeting his outstretched hands, embracing and holding him warmly and promising to always be there for him when he needs her.

Marlin learned to master this technique and used it effectively to overcome his pornography addiction.

Sexual distortion and its restoration

Rudolf Steiner predicted in 1918 that if humanity failed to find the right ideas to further human evolution, several events would occur. One of these is the horrific *distortion of sexuality* that is taking place at every level of our society because people are failing to find love, compassion and empathy for their fellow human being. It is the children, entrusted to our support and care, who are most at risk and who suffer so greatly at the hands of these antihuman distortions of sexuality. The challenge will be to find the courage and strength to stand up in the name of love and compassion for our children and the child within ourselves if we are to resist this scourge to our humanity.[21]

Chapter 11. Addictive Behaviour Patterns

When I observe my inner and outer behaviour patterns, I discover I am hooked into doing things a particular way because they provide me with the greatest comfort, safety and security. I recognise they have been there from my earliest memory and that I myself must have created them as a young child. I realise that all children must do the same as an ingenious psychological means of survival. Who is it that knows how to protect you as a child but forgets to let go when you are grown up? He continues to protect you, restricting you and costing you greatly, including your freedom. I wish to understand how these patterns are set up and how we can overcome them.

—

Up until now we have looked at a range of external agencies that are used by children and youth to satisfy deep unfulfilled needs. We have seen how substances, on the one hand, ingested as food or drink and imbibed in various ways as sanctioned or illicit drugs, can give immediate relief to children who are suffering habitual inner discomfort; on the other, how compulsive engagement in outer activities such as the entertainment media, electronic technology, violence and sexual behaviour, can instantaneously sooth agitation and uneasy feelings that arise in the young person's soul. And because there is nothing else on offer, continuous gratification by this external agency can lead to dependency and ultimately to compulsive addiction.

Internal behaviour dependency

There is however another form of dependency which is habitual and immediately soothing, but which does not require any outside interventions to bring about relief. These are the internal behaviour patterns that are formed in a young child as the soul life responds to environmental impressions and that are instinctively created as the best and safest form of behaviour that will appease his discomfort and satisfy his needs. This requires no prompting by parents, and is created ingeniously by the child himself as he grows up in response to the encounter with his inner and outer environment. Through constant repetition, these behaviour patterns become embedded in the invisible matrix of the psychosomatic continuum as an habitual and reflex response to life. They are usually created in early childhood but, because of their habitual nature, invariably continue throughout the child's life. Because they are so deeply ingrained in subconscious reflex behaviour responses, they will have a major impact on the individual's life.

To the extent that they are repetitive and inflexible behaviour patterns designed to bring relief to a threatening or uncomfortable situation, we may call them addictive behaviour patterns. They provide, like any addictive agency, the comfort and security, in quelling or avoiding pain, because there is no other support to meet the child's deeper inner needs. And even though these actions may cause grave consequences, for the one in need, all that matters for him is the safety and security that this behaviour provides.

The following case studies will illustrate the nature of these behaviour patterns:

Addictive behaviour responses

Ted grew up in a fear-filled environment. His father was prone to violent temper outbursts and when he was drinking, everyone in the family would avoid him, whereas he would look for any reason to create a scene.

Bill grew up afraid of authority, and every encounter with an assertive person or a threatening situation would provoke anxiety and a need to withdraw. He was easily intimidated by more wilful children, terrified of strict teachers and was afraid to face new challenges. He experienced such situations as oppressive and terrifying and discovered for himself that the best way to manage them was to withdraw or avoid them. In later life he was cautious, sensitive and always tense and any challenging situations; examinations or job interviews provoked anxiety.

Thandi was the oldest of six children. Her father laid down the law at home and his authority was firmly imposed by his strictness and his passive aggressive demeanour when his authority was questioned or opposed. If she tried to assert her will, she was firmly rebuked and her father would withdraw his affection. His authority made her feel safe and because she adored him so much, she would do everything possible to please him. She grew up in a male-dominated environment where her younger brothers enjoyed privileges that the sisters did not receive. Thandi learned to regard masculine authority as the power that provided her with security. From early age she gave way to the male-dominated will; she always followed the lead of the boys, never took initiatives of her own and was reluctant to express her own opinions. A common thread throughout her life was to try to win the approval of boys and men; in school, she would do whatever it would take to ingratiate herself with boys and became promiscuous at an early age. She frequently formed relationships with older men and each of her three marriages was to older and assertive men who in different ways dominated and controlled her life. Thandi had learned from the earliest age to submit to the authoritative power of the masculine ego as the best and safest way to avoiding intense inner discomfort.

Sarah was an anxious child. She had parents who were hardworking, high-performing and ambitious for their children. She always wanted to please them and hated above all to disappoint them. If she did things imperfectly, she would berate herself and try to do it better next time. She learned that when things were done according to her high standards she felt happy and secure, whereas when they were done less than perfectly she felt anxious and insecure. This behaviour pattern became a compulsive habit that was driven by obsessive thoughts and feelings of anxiety. In school she was exhausting herself in her efforts to do things in the way it felt right for her. She developed a condition of chronic fatigue that placed severe pressures on her health and her academic ambitions. At the age of twenty-eight she developed breast cancer which resulted in mutilating surgery and recurrent therapeutic interventions. Throughout these challenging situations Sarah continued to act out her inner need for perfectionism, because there was nothing else that could replace her deep inner need for comfort and security.

Bulani learned from the earliest age to become independent. When he was six months old, both parents were working from early morning till late at night. He was cared for by the neighbour, but she could not give him individual attention because she had her own children to look after. He learned to take care of himself and to fight his own battles. He could not rely on anyone to help him when he was in trouble and had to trust in his own abilities to survive in a harsh world. At pre-school he experienced his independence and resilience as a powerful asset and used it to gain friends and control those who threatened his freedom. He soon came up against the boundaries of school life and reacted aggressively to all measures that curtailed his freedom. This led to endless confrontations with teachers and other children, moves to different schools and ultimately expulsion in high school. He found close camaraderie with other township youth who had likewise rebelled against authority and was soon involved in gang-based activities such as drug trafficking and mafia-type protection services. Bulani's powerful need for freedom and independence came from his mistrust of others and the inner feeling that only by maintaining his own freedom could he feel inwardly secure and safe. Even in prison he created his own free spaces and independence by asserting his will as a powerful gang lord.

Our personal experience

If we examine our typical behaviour responses and have the opportunity to study our ingrained behaviour patterns, we will probably find that these inner psychosomatic formations are at the core of many of our life issues. We will discover that these behaviour patterns are so imprinted in our subconscious feeling and behaviour responses that most of the time we don't realise that we are continually acting them out. We begin to realise, sometimes with shock and amazement, that when we are acting out our particular behaviour pattern, *we are assuming a persona that thinks, feels and acts in a certain way that controls our life in much the same way as a drug addict is controlled by a drug.* We can get to know this part of our personality with its unique mindset, and will discover it has a biography that probably begins way back in childhood; we realise that we have continued to act out this persona into the present time because this is the way we learned to feel most secure and we have found no other way of doing it better. We realise that this way of being was established in early childhood as the best means we knew at that time to protect ourselves. An ingenious protector finds the safest and most secure way to survive the inevitable challenges of growing up. Unfortunately the authentic experience of that time becomes entrenched in a habitual behaviour pattern that becomes compulsive and extremely difficult to throw off, even though we are now living in a completely different life experience which in no way coincides with that earlier reality.

Understanding the addictive behaviour pattern

A first step towards overcoming this habituation may be to understand how this addictive patterning comes about. I have found two ways to understand this process: the one is the pneumo-psychosomatic model that Rudolf Steiner presents in his psychosophy lectures of 1910.[1] The other is the psychophonetic counselling process.[2,3,4]

Psychosophy

In accordance with our previous description of the human constitution, we can represent the body-soul-spirit continuum or the pneumo-psychosomatic connection in the following way (see Figure 6):

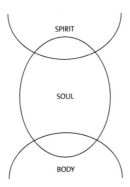

Figure 6. Body-soul-spirit continuum in the human being.

The child's emerging soul exists and develops between the body and spirit. The body is a product of the world of matter, while the spirit is a representative element of the world of spirit. During the child's waking life, his soul life becomes outwardly active and he responds to

223

sense impressions generated by the outer world. These impressions are experienced at the frontier between body and soul through the twelve sense organs that mediate the sense-perceptible world in different ways.[5] The sense impressions set in motion an instant communication between body, soul and spirit where activities such as desires, sensations, feelings, mental pictures and thought processes ultimately lead to actions that are carried out at a physical, psychological or spiritual level. These inner processes can also be activated from within, without outer sensory stimulation.

Let us take the example of Ted who grew up in a very tense home environment where he was frequently experiencing or anticipating his father's violence. Despite his acute fear, Ted is drawn involuntarily to these sensory impressions; his will-based drive to meet the experience and his sensory apparatus have their origin in his bodily processes, impelling him towards the external events. In the moment that he sees his angry father abusing his mother, several events take place instantaneously in his soul life: his body tightens up *(sensation)*, his breathing constricts, he feels anxiety *(feelings)*, an unconscious *memory* of previous events is stirred up and he takes evasive *action* by running to his bedroom and shutting the door. This inner response was set in motion when Ted for the first time experienced these angry scenes as a six-month-old baby. At that stage, he could not run away, but the internal body response *(heightened sensations* and *functional reactivity)* created a pattern of colic, asthma, sleep disturbances and eczematous skin reactions. He voiced his displeasure by crying whenever his father was moody or angry. After this had happened a number of times, the experience of the angry father becomes embedded or memorised into the memory matrix of the bodily system. Thus when Ted experiences another angry person, it immediately evokes a similar response. With further development of his soul life, conscious mental pictures awaken, so that when he hears his father approaching, the unconscious memorised experience of an angry father transforms into a mental picture of a violent scene. He decides that he would be safest inside his room with the door closed. And so runs to his bedroom and shuts the door.

In this manner, a habitual behaviour response is set up as a way of relieving anxiety and creating the maximum sense of security. Later in life, whenever Ted experiences anything threatening, there is an immediate reflex to recoil, to withdraw or to hide. In essence he becomes a small frightened and vulnerable child (see Figure 7).

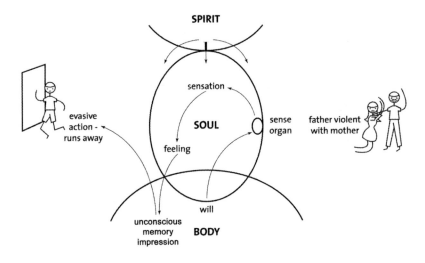

Figure 7. Child taking evasive action to escape from danger.

Psychophonetic counselling

These sessions provide graphic and regular experience of addictive behaviour responses that are invariably established in childhood. A case study will illustrate best the nature of these patterns as well as the way in which they develop.

Ashraf came to see me for a longstanding skin condition that appeared to be related to stressful situations. His boss was constantly berating him for poor quality work, his wife was complaining that he was not earning enough and his children were unhappy that he was not being the best dad because he was always working. Ashraf was not feeling good about himself and he was becoming depressed and unmotivated the more everyone complained about his ineptitudes. He was even having suicidal thoughts.

The picture emerged of a negatively minded person, trapped in a cycle of criticism and despondency which was casting a shadow over his life; any criticism from outside enhanced self-judgment and poor self-image with resultant demotivation and depression. When asked what he wished to do about this situation, Ashraf wanted first to understand how this negative person had become so controlling of his whole life and then

225

to find a way of regaining his confidence.

Recalling an example of his boss criticising him, Ashraf was first asked to become aware of the experience both in his body and in his feelings, and then to gesture how it felt; his body contracted into a tight ball, his head buried in his chest. When he moved out of the position and looked at the form he had created, he could see himself clearly as a young child of five or six years of age, being reprimanded by his father for doing something wrong again, and criticised by his mother for not doing certain duties in the house. He could also see the powerful persona of criticism and judgment that was continuously attacking him. He had copied or imitated this undermining force from his parents and through constant repetition over time, this had become embedded within his own psychosomatic nature. With shock he realised that the personality dynamic that was controlling his life as an adult was no other than this frightened vulnerable child and the harsh critic that had created a self-fulfilling partnership of abuse.

Ashraf had convinced himself that he was not good enough; he was always expecting someone to criticise him and therefore created situations where he would not give his best so that this expectation could be fulfilled. He did this as a reflex response to any critical voice, even his own children and noticed that he felt secure and comfortable in his experience of not doing things well. He had never experienced praise for good work and therefore had no good reason to try to excel. This became an habitual psychological response that had been formed to relieve stress, despite the fact that it created other difficulties for the growing child. He also discovered that there was an internal protector that shielded him from danger by removing him from threatening situations. The addictive behaviour pattern, like all addictions, led to a cycle of negative consequences that could only be unravelled and transformed when the underlying need was recognised.

Internal guardian

There is an internal intelligence within the psyche of every child that is highly attuned on the one hand to the need for safety and security, and on the other to any situation perceived as threatening. Notwithstanding the security and outer care and support that may be present, a child who feels insecure will feel threatened, leading to the internal guardian immediately stepping in to protect him.

Tim who grew up in a fear-filled home environment anticipates danger wherever he goes. He constantly hears the voice of his internal protector telling him to avoid people, back off from potentially threatening situations and to always be extremely cautious.

Thandi who grew up in an aggressive male-dominated home situation, is instructed by her internal guardian to be submissive as the safest way of growing up.

Sarah was constantly trying to live up to the expectation of her parents and was taught by her internal protector to perform to perfection as the best means of creating peace and safety in her life.

Bulani who felt threatened by the world was trained by his internal guardian to be tough, ruthless, mistrustful and aggressive in order to survive.

This protective intelligence is birthed and active during the early and middle phase of the child's development, belonging to that period when his soul life is awakening to the surrounding world. It comes into being at a time when the child feels most sensitive, vulnerable and defenceless and plays an indispensable role in providing the child with some means of inner support and protection. Yet it usually does not disappear when the child feels more secure and confident of himself. This must have to do with the embedding of experiences in the memory matrix of the body, where the patterning of learned behaviour is programmed into the psyche of the child. The internal guardian will therefore continue to protect the vulnerable child as long as it manifests vulnerability. It takes no account of other factors, such as a different current environment, whether this action is of use to the older child or adult or whether it is harmful in other ways to the child. Its mandate is protection of vulnerability and it does this faithfully and with utmost integrity.

Management and caring

From the above case study we can seen how an addictive behaviour pattern, such as poor self-esteem due to a negative self-image, is created in early life and perpetuated throughout the individual's life. The voice of self-judgment may be at the same time the voice of protection of someone who has such feelings of low self-worth. If we follow the case further we can see how this habitualised behaviour pattern can gradually be overcome and transformed in a living and practical way.

> Ashraf could see clearly that his pattern of behaviour was caused by repetitive judgment, blame and criticism and the lack of encouragement, support and praise in his childhood. He could see how a positive loving and supportive influence would have made all the difference. He could also see that such an attitude to himself now would change his negative mindset because the behaviour pattern was as present now as it was then as a child. However to begin with, more was required to break the addictive pattern than simply to change his mental attitude. It is usually not enough to quit cocaine by simply changing one's mental attitude. If a positive support had been present for the child, it would have been a living physical and psychological experience for him and not purely an intellectual one. The child would have had to experience directly the positive value of encouragement and praise. Therefore now a positive, supportive character needs to be present who will engage on a regular basis with this negatively minded child and through ongoing interaction convince him that he is good enough, that he can do good things and there were many good reasons why it is worth while trying hard to do one's best. Ashraf was able firstly to imagine such a character, then embody it in himself and then act it out in life. Through constant repetition over several weeks, he was able to introduce motivation and confidence into his life. This surprised most of all himself, and the positive responses from his boss, wife and children were further reasons to maintain his new-found attitude to life.

It should be abundantly clear from what has been described thus far that these behaviour patterns are deeply entrenched in the body-soul continuum. They need to be clearly recognised for what they are as addictive psychosomatic reflex activities that provided security at a time when the child was extremely vulnerable and which have become imprinted into the body and psyche through constant repetition. This is a fixed functional and psychological pattern that cannot be erased by wishful thinking. It can only be changed through recognising the inner child's deep insecurity and helping him in an active way to overcome his fears. This may be done by offering him an alternative that not only provides adequate security, but also gives him the opportunity of learning himself to manage his fear. An active and living relationship with the inner child will need to develop, whereby regular conversations and interactions can take place to increase his confidence and security. As this grows, real live opportunities need to be created to show him how to overcome his fear and to break his cycle of dependency on his internal protector.

It is probable that every individual carries within them ingrained behaviour patterns of this kind as a normal adaptive process of survival. They almost certainly served the child well at the time they were established and may continue to provide safety and security for the rest of the person's life. However, like any addictive process these benefits inevitably come with a price. They invariably trap the individual in a cycle of dependency that will curtail his freedom and limit his potential for his fullest expression and fulfilment in life.

If one wishes to learn to manage this dependency, the fundamental steps for managing any addictive process will need to be put in place:

- Firstly, the addictive pattern has to be clearly recognised.
- Secondly, a living connection has to be made with the internal characters who control one's life.
- Then steps have to be taken to dehabitualise the ingrained psychosomatic pattern by providing a better alternative.
- Finally, this has to be reinforced consistently and repetitively until this new habit pattern is taken up by the unconscious psychosomatic programming.

In my experience, the first level of deconditioning will require about four weeks, the time generally needed for new habits to be acquired; new skills such as riding a bicycle or training a particular unused muscle usually requires this period of time as the first phase of new skill development. In this process, a focused force of will and energy is needed to work on that part of our constitution that carries habits and memory. In astrological and intuitive science, this latter part, known as the life body, has a relationship with the moon; the self-directing power of the *I* or higher *Self* where choice and resolutions are at work, is represented by the sun. The moon, which takes approximately twenty-nine days to orbit the sun and to return to its original position in relation to the sun, is irradiated each day by the sun and moves daily into a different relationship with the earth. In like manner, the resonating life body, which stores all experiences as vibrational qualities, is imprinted daily with new self-directed impressions so that after about four weeks it too has returned to its original position. In this time it has learned to recognise the new pattern and can communicate this to the physical and soul bodies with which it interfaces.

For permanent transformation of this behaviour pattern, however, this deconditioning process needs to continue for the best part of twelve months. This is comparable to the movement of the sun through the twelve constellations of the zodiac, continually irradiating the moon. Thereafter, a new directing force will be in place, one that has been consciously chosen and created. Although vestiges of the old habit may still remain, they will, by and large, be subject to the care and guidance of this new power, which will open the way to new life opportunities.

The struggle of our times

From the moment one discovers an internal addictive behaviour pattern and chooses to transform it, a struggle develops between two forces: one that originates in the past, that is based on fear or doubt or hatred and that would bind one into dependency and addiction; and another that comes from the future, that chooses rather to work with courage, creativity and love and that carries the impulse to be free.

This is the challenge that has to be faced in all addictions, the battle between dependency that belongs to the past, and freedom that strives towards the future. This theme will be continued in the next chapter.

Chapter 12. The Battle for the Human Soul

I hear the call for freedom in the human soul; it resonates in the quest for independence, for self-authority and for emancipation from dependency and enslavement of all kinds. Yet we seem to live in dependency and bondage, we carry it into our lives from the past; indeed we ourselves create it in our childhood. There are forces in the world that, through self-interest and egoism, are invested in promoting servitude in others. Vulnerability creates dependency and children who are the most vulnerable are most at risk of becoming dependent and losing their freedom.

I wish to know more about this battle for freedom. I need to understand the dependent one, the enslaving one, as well as the free spirit. Then I will be in the best position to guide the children in my care to freedom.

—

The struggle for freedom

A less well-known version of an ancient Greek legend tells of Persephone, the daughter of Demeter, an innocent maiden who is seduced in subtle and devious ways by Pluto, the god of the underworld. She is taken by him to Hades, into the realm of the dead, or the underworld, where she goes through dramatic encounters with despair, death, powerlessness and suicide. Pluto wants her to drink the juice of the pomegranate fruit so that she will forget her previous life and become the Queen of the Dead.

To begin with she resists, but gradually she succumbs to his fascinating powers and is about ready to drink the dark red juice when Triptolemos, a young prince, arrives on the scene. He heard of Persephone's fate from Demeter, the mother of Persephone who, disguised as an old widow, is grieving the loss of her daughter. He chooses to rescue Persephone rather than claim the crown of his father who has just died. With Hecate's help he breaks into Pluto's realm and calls on Persephone to remind her where she came from. In that moment she drops the cup from her lips and is able to leave Hades with her new prince.

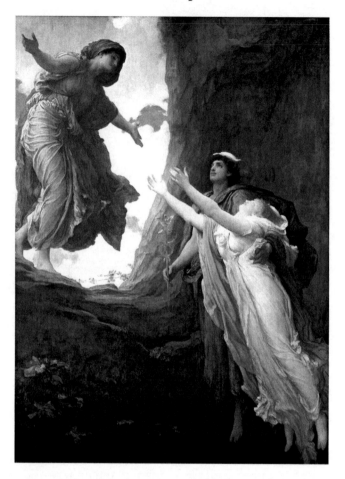

Figure 8. The Return of Persephone, by Frederic Leighton (1891).

Anyone who has tried to counter the grip that dependency of any kind has on their inner life will know that a battle for freedom is being waged in the human soul. On the one side there is the partnership of dependency where a false prophet offers, to someone in need, comfort and security, but requires the needy one to be forever in bondage to him. Pluto offers to Persephone the power of a queendom, but she will forever have to reign within his underworld kingdom. On the other side there is Triptolemos, the messenger of freedom, the one who represents the free Self, who wishes to guide the soul to make choices and take action in accordance with her true nature. Triptolemos reveres the true nature of Persephone and makes whatever sacrifices are needed to ensure that she can express her true nature and rightful destiny in a land of freedom.

If we are to understand why children and adolescents are most at risk in becoming dependent on addictive substances, agencies or behaviours, and why most addictions in adult life have their origins in childhood or adolescence, we shall need to consider two themes: on the one hand, the hazards of growing up; on the other, the vulnerable nature of the developing psyche.

Hazards of growing up

Consider what modern day children have to face growing up in the twenty-first century. They face a minefield of potential hazards that threaten every phase of their existence.

In the womb, the embryo and foetus are completely dependent on the maternal environment for its survival and wellbeing and will be subject to all the physical, chemical, nutritional and psychological impressions to which the mother is exposed. Though the foetus may be well protected within the mother's body, it can still be harmed by external influences, for instance what the mother eats or drinks, the drugs she takes or the kind of life she leads. Indeed its life can be summarily terminated if the parents or other stakeholders regard its presence as too much trouble to allow it to continue to live and be born.

From the moment of birth, the child may be exposed to the rigours of a harsh external environment: immunisation, chemical medicines, toxic pollutants, nutritional stresses, violence and abuse in the home and society.

In later life the child may be subjected to the toxic and addictive effects of the sanctioned drugs – caffeine, nicotine and alcohol – as well as the wide range of illicit substances, discussed in Chapters 5 and 6.

She will engage intimately with the seductive allure of electronic technology and mass media and be exposed to sensational information and horrifying images that are completely unsuitable for the growing child. She will experience the violence, cruelty, depravity and inhumanness and the many other dark forces that inhabit the human souls of people around her. She will also come to face this within her own soul.

Development of the soul

In Chapter 1, we traced the development of the child's soul life from birth to adulthood. In the first seven years, the soul is submerged in bodily processes and expresses itself through bodily functions. It is not yet able to express itself independently of the body. An infant suckling happily on its mother's breast shows its pleasure in the rhythmic movement of the fingers and toes; displeasure and discomfort will be expressed in intestinal cramping or other bodily dysfunctions. The soul life is still intricately bound up with bodily processes so that it cannot act without affecting in some way the function of the body. During this period, the soul primarily serves the needs and functions of the body, working strongly through the soul functions of will impulses and sense perception. Its delicate nature, like a vulnerable embryo, is protected by the body, which itself needs the continuous care and protection of parents and other carers.

With the change of teeth a part of the soul life begins to free itself from the body and awakens to its own independent nature. Feelings – the heart centre of the soul – begin to awaken without impacting on or interfering with physiological function. This highly sensitive and most personal part of the soul opens itself innocently to the surrounding world, exposing itself ever more to the unpredictable vagaries of external life. For the first few years there is still an instinctive need to remain close to the protection of parents and other family members who provide a natural protective sheath as the child makes the transition into an independent social life. But as the child approaches puberty, there is more and more need to be free of the security provided by parents and family and to replace it with the community of friends and comrades. It is understandable therefore that through peer pressure and social identification, children from the age of around ten will inevitably become exposed to the substances and activities that can lead to dependency and addiction.

Puberty is a critical milestone in the development of the soul. As described in Chapter 2, the teenager awakens to new-found powers, physically, sexually, emotionally and intellectually. Despite her new-found independence, the adolescent secretively will still feel the need for moral support and it is essential that the adults in the family, in the school community and as friends and mentors, are actively present, as a balancing factor in her life. For if her psychological needs have not been properly addressed throughout the preceding growth periods, and there is no one who notices her dissatisfaction and distress, then the awakened power of will, desires, feelings and independence of thinking can draw the adolescent towards those addictive agencies we have described above.

As the continuum of body, soul and spirit develops through these three cycles of seven years, three important formations are established in the growing child that will influence the susceptibility of the child to addictive behaviour. These internal supersensible structures are the constitution, the temperament and the character.

Formation of the constitution, temperament and character

In the first seven years, the *physical constitution* will be established.[1] We can differentiate three main types, a *head* type, a *chest* type and a *metabolic* type, depending on which principal organ centre predominates. The head type is characterised by a predominant neuro-sensory system, which may manifest as either an introverted *cerebral* subtype or a more extraverted *sensory* subtype. In the chest type, the chest region predominates where the feelings in the *respiratory* subtype tend to be very changeable, while in the *cardiac* subtype they are usually intense in nature. The metabolic type has a powerful metabolism where the *digestive* subtype tends to be adaptable and placid, whereas the *limb* subtype has a strong physique and strength of will.

We have seen how the preferential development of the will and sensory functions during this period opens the trusting child to all the impressions of the outer world. Innocently and without the ability to guard or protect herself, she will imprint these impressions, both the positive and the negative, into her life body, from where their resonance will vibrate into her bodily as well as her soul life. This, as we have seen is the basis of *imitation*, the fundamental power of learning in the young child.

These impressions will be imbibed qualitatively differently according to the child's constitutional makeup. Thus the sensory subtype will take in so many impressions, she may be flooded by them and will find it difficult to be aware of them all and to name them clearly; the cerebral subtype will shape the impressions cognitively but may lack feelings or the impulse to act on them; the cardiac and respiratory subtype will experience them more on the feeling level and may have difficulty articulating or expressing them; the digestive subtype will need time to digest her sensory experiences and may be slow cognitively, while the limb subtype may tend to act out impulsively what she perceives.

In the second seven year period, with the awakening of the feelings, the *temperament,* which expresses the evolving life processes, is established constitutionally.[2] There are four main temperaments, a legacy of the time of Hippocrates, the ancient Greek physician, and which are connected with the four elements. The *melancholic* temperament is weighed down by the heaviness and compactness of the *earth* element; the *phlegmatic* temperament flows in the ease and comfort of the *water* element; the *sanguine* temperament floats in the lightness and volatility of the *air* element; the *choleric* temperament is activated by the heat and power of the *warmth* element. One can imagine how these temperaments will influence the sensory perceptions, the inner imagination, cognition, feelings, emotions and actions of the child, laying down the formative elements of the personality still to be formed. Thus a melancholic child will tend to be more introverted, cautious and anxious, whereas a choleric child will be confident and fearless; a sanguine child will experience life lightly, whereas the phlegmatic will be ponderous and avoid difficulties.

It is only in the third seven year period, as the soul awakens out of its slumber within the bodily processes and the soul faculty of thinking comes to the fore, that the *personality* or *character* is formed.[3] This is a highly complex construction where the impressions of the outer world, coloured by the constitution and temperament, meet the inner disposition shaped by pre-birth experiences. In my book *Awakening to Child Health,* I describe seven character types that emerge in the march to adulthood. There is the self-orientated individual type which contrasts strongly with the imitating, following type; the organised centred type differs sharply from the connecting mobile type; and the active masculine type stands in contrast to the receptive feminine type; finally there is the harmonious balanced type which carries elements of all the other types in a harmonious balance.

Within these different personality types, a cast of characters emerges, coming into being or fortified in response to the inner experiences of the growing child. Every one of these characters are real personalities who think, feel and behave in very definite ways. They do not simply arise out of the woodwork, nor do they randomly appear in response to some environmental stimulus. They come into being because someone invited them, someone who knows they are needed for some good reason.

Who is this invisible director who chooses the cast best able to serve his life work?

Awakening of the I

If we listen closely to our inner life, we will discern the above mentioned host of inner characters who can or cannot do this or that, who like or hate this or that, who want or reject this or that. However, beyond all these varied characters and their sometimes frenzied activity, we may discern another presence that directs this inner life, that holds the balance between all the different voices and intentions, that can make choices and resolutions and takes actions that will determine the direction of life. This is a power that can deny the life of desire and contain the sea of emotions. It stands not for black or white, for comfort and pleasure, but for what is good and true. It is the *I* or *Self* that lives as the core being of every individual. Can we observe the presence of this core being in the developmental process?

In the third year of life, most children become aware of themselves as a person separate from other persons and for the first time, Sarah calls herself *I* and no longer Sarah. This little word is the only word in all languages that is used to refer to oneself and cannot be used to refer to anyone or anything else. It must relate to an aspect of self that stands at the very centre of one's being. As such it must have central significance for every part of the human constitution, for body, soul and spirit and must be active in the entire growth process of the child to adulthood. It cannot be regarded as a product of the body but has to be seen as a source or wellspring of our life here on earth.

Whereas our soul life is visible to us in some part of its nature, as our personal kingdom of inner experience, our *I* is mostly hidden to our consciousness, flashing up into our awareness only in moments of intuition. It is a profound mystery that we are hardly aware of that part of our being that expresses our eternal and most essential nature. We may see it flashing through the development of the child in fleeting moments: when the child names something in a way that is completely unique to that child; in the first precious moment when the child calls herself *I*; when conscious choices are made and clear views are expressed; in the tenth year, when the child experiences the intense loneliness and separation from her childhood protection as a kind of fall from paradise; and again at around fifteen years, when the adolescent feels a longing for home and for finding a hero; and then when she begins the quest to know 'who I am, who you are and where I am going'; with eighteen there is someone who feels the power to meet the challenges of life alone and who is able to orientate herself in the world; in the following two to three years, life choices and decisions are often made and actions taken that will determine future outcomes. At the age of around twenty one, a self-contained individual emerges who can take hold of her life and destiny and can for the most part take care of herself.

In this period of twenty-one years, three times seven years, the body and soul have been prepared and shaped as suitable instruments for carrying the awakened *I* into the world. The *I*, as core member of our being, is always present as the body and soul mature, and like the light which shapes the eye and then uses the eye as the perfect organ for seeing, so does the *I* shape the body and the soul to create the best organs for manifesting its work in the world.

Forces of darkness

We are all well aware that there are elements within us that make us smaller than we know we are or would like to be. We would like to be strong or brave but something within prevents us from being this and makes us feel weak or fearful. 'You are crazy to think you are strong enough!' 'You are not brave enough to act out your convictions!' Voices of negativity constantly undermine, accuse and condemn us, making us feel ashamed and guilty. 'You're stupid and pathetic!' – 'You are the cause of all your problems!' – 'You should be ashamed of yourself to have such an opinion.' We would like to become something or do something, but something within stops us from becoming it or doing it. Ashraf wanted to be a good husband and father but his doubt, fear or self-judgment prevented him from becoming what he wanted to be.

When we learn how to turn the light on within the psyche, we discover the very colourful and active troupe of characters, described above, who live in this twilight world of the soul, waiting for their cue to act out their role in our life drama. And as we survey this internal drama, it becomes very clear that the psyche is inhabited by forces that are not only benevolent and expansive, but also harmful and restrictive in their nature. These latter forces will have a profound effect on the physical and psychological development of the child.

How do these characters land up in our most intimate inner life and why have characters been invited that are clearly harmful to our wellbeing?

The origin of negative forces

When we explore the inner terrain further, we discover that these personae have been created in response to a wide range of factors.

The first provisional soul structure is formed on the one hand by the outer life – the environment, family life, school life, society, religion and culture; on the other by the inner life – the inner disposition from the past, hereditary influences, the constitution and temperament. Within this configuration, the awakening soul of the child meets the harsh reality of the outer world and in this cauldron of emerging soul life, the creation of these characters take place.

The genius within the child knows instinctively what persona is needed in order to best navigate the difficult waters. With regular prompting from outside, and knowing the internal inclinations and predispositions, the inner director takes up these cues and fashions the right character to meet the life situation which destiny dictates to the child.

Thandi who grows up from day one in a male-dominated family creates for herself a passive and submissive character who offers her maximum safety and security. This character will give form and direction to the unfolding of her receptive feminine personality type. It will receive a further colouring by her sanguine nature and by her respiratory constitution.

Bulani on the other hand absorbs the powerful authority of his father and fashions for himself a dominating masculine personality. This character best satisfies his need to be in control and his choleric temperament and limb constitution will further shape his personality.

The battleground of the soul

In this way, the soul becomes inhabited by a variety of different characters whose nature may be very different and indeed contradictory. For instance, Thandi may outwardly exhibit her submissive character, but inwardly she carries a rebellious persona who would love to defy the male authority in her home. This character she creates as the inner counterweight to the tensions and resentments that arise in her by always submitting to the dominant male authority in her home.

The soul becomes the personal home for an array of personae, all of whom are given a place and a role in the life of the one who chooses and constructs their nature. As we have said there are personae who are expansive, open and forward-looking in their nature; there are others that are constrictive, closed and backward-looking in their intentions and actions. A character who is terrified to perform in front of the class is harassed by another who tells her what a coward she is. The bully who beats up other children as a way of releasing the tension from her own abusive home life feels ashamed and guilty for what she has done.

The soul inevitably becomes the battlefield for horrendous inner battles between opposing characters. And because the soul is a receptacle – for the body on the one side, and for the spirit on the other – it will also absorb all manner of negative influences coming from these regions.

The body which houses the unconscious will, forces of instinct, drives and desires, can unleash into the soul life the most powerful violent forces which will be taken up by the characters that reside in the human soul. Forces that live in the power of matter, in the bodily nature, working through the unconscious will, can wreak havoc in the awakening soul life of the adolescent person. They are nature forces – like hurricanes, earthquakes and tsunamis – that can be unleashed when the right conditions prevail. The drive to bully another child, the desire for a drug that gives physical prowess or the power acquired by computer games, are driven largely by these forces that belong to this unconscious region. These forces can receive ammunition from all the external and internal addictive agencies we have described in this book.

On the other side, the emerging intellect and the growing independence of rational thinking give new meaning and direction to the awakening soul. The growing intellect is gullible and highly impressionable to influences that address the youth's most pressing issues. These come in many different guises, in the role models of their heroes, in music and song, in advertising, movies, and through peer pressure. Young people will take up these messages and create plausible and convincing arguments for carrying out any manner of atrocious deeds. They will be able to justify any reckless behaviour – binge drinking, sexual promiscuity, cutting themselves and even suicide – as right things to be done. These forces coming from the spiritual side also thrust themselves into the arena of the soul, sometimes with devastating consequences (see Figure 9).

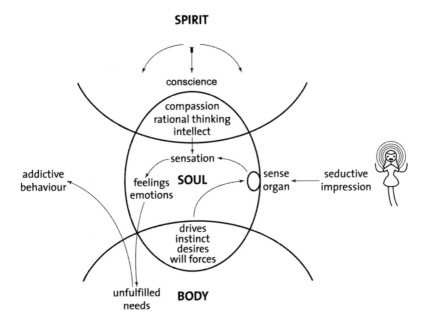

Figure 9. Seductive impression on the human being.

The battle

It is within this context that we can place the pandemic phenomena of child and adolescent addictions. The child who is exposed to addictive agencies is seduced by forces that are seemingly beyond her control. She feels alone, without care or protection, because some basic need within her has not been met. This, as we have seen, lies at the root of the addictive tendency. This need is like a desperately hungry person who will be drawn towards some food gratification that will give at least temporary relief to the deep discomfort caused by the hunger. But at the same time, from deep within the child's being, there is resistance to giving herself over to a force of gratification that she knows is innately false and harmful.

The stage is set for a terrible battle of wills within the tender growing soul of the child. The needy hungry child seeks to appease her hunger. A saviour in the form of food, a drug, mass media, a computer or a particular soul character, gives her the comforting food that relieves her hunger. He does not tell her that this gratification will be temporary and that she will continue to be needy; nor that she will need more and more food to satisfy her hunger so that she becomes ever more desperate. She is not told that she will become dependent like a trapped and submissive slave or that her health will decline, leading to the emergence of many other problems, including a new character called *Dis-ease;* nor will he warn her that her life and family will be thrown into chaos, confusion and untold suffering, creating other negative characters of grief, guilt, shame, poor self-esteem, fear and many others that will cast further shadows over her life. This false prophet has only one intent, to provide relief to the hungry soul and becomes like all the many others in the child's soul, a real live character.

Other voices emerge amid the roars and cries of the battlefield: the voice of caution attempts to warn her of the dangers; conscience tries to change her course of direction; compassion for her suffering and that of her parents endeavours to loosen the addictive grip; and reason tries its best to persuade her to seek another route of action. They all stand ready to oppose the power of the seductive saviour.

It is a battle for control of the human soul, for if the needy child can be enticed to drink the draught of the pomegranate juice, and no other force can break apart this alliance of dependency, then all the forces of the soul will have to submit to the authority of the Lord of the Underworld.

The quest for freedom

There is only one power that can save the child's soul and prevent it from sliding into the abyss of dependency and bondage. *It is the will to be a free individual.* Something within the child must want to be free and to galvanise all those forces of the soul that can help wrest the child from the dark forces of seductive dependency. This power can only come from that free space in the child's being that exists beyond body, soul and spirit, that sphere of inner authority and pure activity, in which the choice maker, the integrator, the intuitive, the source and wellspring of our being, the human *I*, resides.

The *I* in the growing child has not yet awakened or is only gradually emerging as a conscious guiding power. It needs to be represented by adult individuals whose *I* have awakened and who can help take charge of the war raging in the child's soul.

Hecate and Demeter will need to guide the youthful Triptolemos to penetrate consciously the dark world of Hades and to actively intervene to break the spell that Pluto has over Persephone. He carries the free spirit that Persephone needs to take herself back into the world of life and light.

It is only from a free space that the endangered youth can gain a clear picture of her neediness and her dependency, and it is only in freedom that she can then choose the right means of caring for her needy child. This may require, as has been illustrated in several case studies, that she finds or creates within herself a character of compassion, of strength, of understanding, of a mother or father, friend or mentor. Through freedom, she then can actively and continuously intervene to break the seductive charm of the false saviour that has created the dependency and addictive tendency.

When, with empathy and insight, we survey the human tragedy caused by childhood and adolescent addiction, we will realise that these children and youth are facing an enormous battle against the most powerful anti-human forces.

These are forces that have been active in the human soul from time immemorial. At a time when the common human being did not yet possess the consciousness of independent thinking, there were divinities, priests and kings that guided humanity like a shepherd guiding his flock. These were, to begin with, benevolent forces that nurtured and cared for the human race. Then humanity came of age and broke away from the rules and regulations of the elders that directed the will of the people and kept them in bondage.

Those forces of the past that would strive to maintain the old order of the world and would block the independent quest for freedom become anti-forces of a humanity that must progress towards the future. The banner that this progressive humanity carries into the future is that of *freedom*. This is the great struggle of our times, the struggle between forces that hold back the free will of the spirit and those forces that seek through free initiative to manifest the free spirit.

This battle is playing itself out both on the outer world stage as well as within the inner life of the soul. History depicts this struggle of nations and societal groups to be free of domination, and at the present time we are seeing another powerful surge within some Arab nations to free themselves from the subjugation of old dynasties. Every generation in most societies carries a wave of renewal that manifests through new initiatives and new ways of behaving; through new ideology, dress code, music, dance, art forms, and many other innovations, we witness the indomitable power of the human spirit to be free. We see this quest for freedom also in the adolescent journey to independence as an adult.

The impulse for all outer action, whether it be nations at war or peace, within societal groups and communities or in the initiatives and actions of individuals, originates within the individual human psyche. It is here that the struggle for freedom is always present, the freedom to break away from the old and forge the new, to move from a dark and restricted view of life to a light and expansive one, to liberate oneself from dependency and discover freedom and independence. This struggle, as we have seen, is nowhere more evident and more challenging than in the child or adolescent caught up in the web of addiction. It is the time-honoured challenge to become a free human being.

It is only the will to be a free individual and the action that follows that can safeguard the integrity and autonomy of the human being. It is this power that needs to take root in the youthful soul trapped in her addictive behaviour. Adults who have awakened in their will to be free can be of great help to these youth. We have seen that it is possible with a little guidance and coaching for anyone to explore the living drama of the human soul and to discover all the characters engaged in this struggle for freedom. When we survey this drama, we are in the open space to express our free will and to oppose those anti-human forces that would limit our potential.

Those of us who cherish this ideal and awaken to this power of freedom will have deep empathy and compassion for children and youth whose will forces have been sub-ordinated to the will of an addictive agency. We shall be empowered through our own liberated experience, our compassion and empathy, our deep insight and conscious awareness, and our active will, to support the dependent youth and to help her discover her independent power to become a free and autonomous human being. This way we stand the chance of safeguarding for the child and her future life, what her *I* claims as her natural birthright – *her freedom.*

It is up to us to make sure that this happens.

Notes

FOREWORD

1. As an expression-based counselling method, psychophonetics extends the client-centred conversational approach to psychotherapy with non-verbal expressive modalities of body awareness, gesture and movement, visualisation and use of the sounds of human speech. This allows rapid access to deep psycho-emotional layers of experience. It is a short-term counselling-coaching process that encourages people to take responsibility for their own healing, transformation and development. It supports relationship development, sexuality, parenthood, vocation, creative and artistic expression and spirituality. It facilitates effective recovery from a wide range of psycho-emotional problems, including addiction, depression, anxiety, trauma, abuse and dysfunctional behaviour patterns. It can also be used actively in any system of holistic or integrated medicine in the healing of a range of physical and psychosomatic conditions.

2. Goldberg, R. (2010) *Awakening to Child Health Part I* (second edition), Hawthorn Press, Stroud, UK.

3. Goldberg, R. (2007–8) Articles written for *South African Journal of Natural Medicine.*

CHAPTER 1

1. Maslow, A.H. (1943) 'A Theory of Human Motivation,' *Psychological Review,* 50 (4): pp.370–96.

2. Maslow, A.H. (1954) *Motivation and Personality,* Harper, New York, p.236.

3. Steiner, R. (1921/1981) *Study of Man,* Rudolf Steiner Press, London.

4. Steiner, R. (1910/1997) *An Outline of Esoteric Science,* Anthroposophic Press, Hudson, NY.

CHAPTER 2

1. Goldberg, R. *Awakening to Deep Experience:* www.drraoulgoldberg.com, www.syringahealth.co.za.

2. Goldberg, R. (2010) *Awakening to Child Health Part I* (seond edition), Hawthorn Press, Stroud, UK.

3. Tagar, Y. (1986–2006) *Psychophonetics: A Collection of Articles, IAPP:* www.psychophonetics.co..au /pages/articles.html.

4. Steele, R. (2011) *Holistic Counseling and Psychotherapy: Stories and Insights from Practice,* Lindisfarne Books, USA.

5. Steele, R. 'A hermeneutic phenomenological study of/in transformation: An embodied and creative exploration of therapeutic change through Psychophonetics psychotherapy.' PhD thesis, Edith Cowan University, Western Australia.

6. Miller, N.S., Giannini, A.J. (1990) 'The disease model of addiction: a biopsychiatrist's view,' *J. Psychoactive Drugs,* 22.

7. Feltenstein, M.W. (2008 May) 'The neurocircuitry of addiction: an overview,' *British Journal of Pharmacology,* 154 (2): pp.261–74.

8. Kalivas P.W., Volkow N.D. (2005) 'The neural basis of addiction: a pathology of motivation and choice,' *American Journal of Psychiatry,* 162 (8): pp.1403–13.

9. Arias-Carrión, O., Pöppel, E. (2007) 'Dopamine, learning, reward-seeking behaviour,' *Act Neurobiol Exp,* 67 (4): pp.481–88.

10. Searle, J.R. (1992) *The Rediscovery of the Mind,* MIT Press, USA.

11. McCauley, K.T. *Is Addiction a Disease?* www.instituteforaddiction-study.com.

CHAPTER 3

1. Harwood, A.C. (1982) *The Recovery of Man in Childhood,* Anthroposophic Press, Spring Valley, NY.

2. Harwood, A.C. (1967) *The Way of a Child,* Rudolf Steiner Press, London.

3. Goldberg, R. (2010) *Awakening to Child health Part I,* (second edition), Hawthorn Press, Stroud.

4. Internal Training Manual of Persephone Institute of Psychophonetics.

5. Syringa Integrated Health Centre: www.syringahealth.co.za.

6. Recommended reading:

Vogt, F. (2002) *Addiction's Many Faces,* Hawthorn Press, Stroud, UK.

Dunselman, R. (1995) *In Place of the Self,* Hawthorn Press, Stroud, UK.

Kaplan & Sadock (1998) *Synopsis of Psychiatry* (eighth edition), Lippencott, Williams & Wilkins, Baltimore, Maryland, USA.

Lievegoed, B. (1987) *Phases of Childhood,* Floris Books, Edinburgh

Steiner, R. (1975) *Education of the Child,* Rudolf Steiner Press, London.

CHAPTER 4

1. Kaplan & Sadock (1998) *Synopsis of Psychiatry,* eighth edition, Lippencott, Williams & Wilkins, Baltimore, Maryland, USA.

2. Kerwin, M.L.E. (1999) 'Empirically supported treatments in pediatric psychology: Severe feeding problems,' *Journal of Pediatric Psychology,* 24 (3), pp.193–214.

3. Robin, A.L., Gilroy, M., Dennis, A.B. (1998) 'Treatment of Eating Disorders in Children and Adolescents,' *Clinical Psychology Review,* 18 (4): pp.421–46.

4. Serdula, M.K., Ivery, D., Coates, R.J., Freedman, D.S., Williamson, D.F., Byers, T. (2002) *Do Obese Children Become Obese Adults? A Review of the Literature,* National Centre for Chronic Disease Prevention, Atlanta, USA.

5. Lobstein, T., Baur, L., Uauy, R. (2004) 'Obesity in children and young people: a crisis in public health,' *Obes Rev,* 5, supplement 1: pp.4–85.

6. NHS: The Information Centre for Health and Social Care (2011) *Statistics on obesity, England:* www.ic.nhs.ukww.

7. Wang, Y., Lobstein, T. (2006) 'Worldwide trends in childhood overweight and obesity.' *International Journal of Pediatric Obesity,* Vol.1, No.1, pp.11–25.

8. Welsh, J.A., Sharma, A., Cunningham, S.A., Vos, M.B. (2011) 'Consumption of Added Sugars and Indicators of Cardiovascular Disease Risk Among US Adolescents,' *Circulation,* 123: pp.249–57.

9. Szabo, C.P. (1997) 'Abnormal Eating Attitudes in Secondary School Girls in South Africa – a preliminary study,' *SA Med J,* 4, supplement, pp.524-26, 528-30.

10. Klump, K.L., Miller, K.B., Keel, P.K., McGue, M., Iacono, W.G. (May 2001) 'Genetic and environmental influences on anorexia nervosa syndromes in a population-based twin sample,' *Psychological Medicine,* 31 (4): pp.737–40.

11. Kortegaard, L.S., Hoerder, K., Joergensen, J, Gillberg, C., Kyvik, K.O. (Feb 2001) 'A preliminary population-based twin study of self-reported eating disorder,' *Psychological Medicine,* 31 (2): pp.361–65.

12. Derenne, J.L., Beresin, E.V. (May-June 2006) 'Body Image, Media, and Eating Disorders,' *Acad Psychiatry,* 30: pp.257-61.

13. Szabo, C.P. (April 1997) 'Factors influencing eating attitudes in secondary-school girls in South Africa – a preliminary study,' *SAMJ,* Volume 87, No.4.

14. Pike, K.M., Rodin, J. (1991) 'Mothers, daughters and disordered eating,' *Journal of Abnormal Psychology,* 97: pp.198–204.

15. Mukai, T. *et al.* (1994) 'Eating attitudes and weight preoccupation among female high school students in Japan,' *J Child Psychol Psychiatry*, 35: pp.677–88S.

16. Goldberg, R. (2006) 'Eating Disorders in Children,' *Natural Medicine*, Issue 23.

17. Rayworth, B.B., Wise, L.A., Harlow, B.H. (2004) 'Child Abuse and Risk of Eating Disorders in Women,' *Epidemiology*, Volume 15, No.3, pp.271–78.

18. The programme offered by the Syringa Child Clinic – a holistic child clinic for sensitive children and adolescents and their reactive syndromes, located at the Syringa Integrated Health Centre in Cape Town – offers an holistic approach to each individual case.

CHAPTER 5

1. Rang, Dale & Ritter (1995) *eds.*, *Pharmacology*, third edition, Churchill Livingstone, UK.

2. Livingstone Black, Rosemary (2010-10-19) 'Boozy energy drink Four Loko – aka 'Blackout in a Can' – banned from N.J. college,' *Daily News* (New York).

3. *Caffeine Content of Food and Drugs*, (2009-08-03) Nutrition Action Health Newsletter, Centre for Science in the Public Interest.

4. *Caffeine Content of Drinks*, Energy Fiend. (2011-03-04): www.energy-fiend.com/the-caffeine-database

5. Knight, C.A., Knight, I., Mitchell, D.C., *et al.* (2004) 'Beverage caffeine intake in US consumers and subpopulations of interest: estimates from the Share of Intake Panel survey,' *Food and Chemical Toxicology*, 42, 1923–1930.

6. Barone, J.J., Roberts, H.R. (14 August 1995) *Caffeine Consumption*, National Soft Drink Association.

7. Valek, M., Laslavic, B. & Laslavic, Z. (2004) 'Daily caffeine intake among Osijek High School students: questionnaire study,' *Croatian Medical Journal*, 45, 72–75.

8. Pollak, C.P. & Bright, D. (2003) 'Caffeine consumption and weekly sleep patterns in US seventh-, eighth-, and ninth-graders,' *Pediatrics*, 111, pp.42–46.

9. Hering-Hanit, R. & Gadoth, N. (2003) 'Caffeine-induced headache in children and adolescents,' *Cephalalgia*, 23, 332–335.

10. Kaplan & Sadock's *Synopsis of Psychiatry* (1998) Eighth Edition, Lippencott, Williams & Wilkins, Baltimore, Maryland, USA.

11. Bernstein, G. A., Carroll, M.E., Thuras, P.D., *et al.* (2002) 'Caffeine

dependence in teenagers,' *Drug and Alcohol Dependence,* 66, pp.1–6.

12. Daly, J.W., Fredholm, B.B. (1998) 'Caffeine – an atypical drug of dependence,' *Drug and Alcohol Dependence,* 51: pp.199–206.

13. Centers for Disease Control and Prevention (CDC) (2009). 'Cigarette smoking among adults and trends in smoking cessation,' 58 (44): pp.1227–32.

14. Stanton, W. (1992) 'A longitudinal study of the influence of parents and friends on children's initiation of smoking,' *Journal of Applied Developmental Psychology,* 13 (4): pp.423–34.

15. Chassin, L., Presson, C., Rose, J., Sherman, S.J., Prost, J. (2002) 'Parental Smoking Cessation and Adolescent Smoking,' *Journal of Pediatric Psychology,* 27 (6): pp.485–96.

16. Charlesworth A, Glantz S.A. (2005) 'Smoking in the movies increases adolescent smoking: a review,' *Pediatrics,* Dec 116 (6): pp.1516–28.

17. Centers for Disease Control and Prevention (CDC) (2007) 'High School Students Who Tried to Quit Smoking Cigarettes,' *Morbidity and Mortality Weekly Report,* 58 (16): pp.428-31.

18. Wood, P.B. (2008) 'Role of central dopamine in pain and analgesia,' *Expert Rev Neurother,* 8 (5): pp.781–97.

19. Pich, E.M., Pagliusi, S.R.,Tessari, M., Talabot-Ayer, D., Hooft Van Huijsduijnen, R., Chiamulera, C. (1997) 'Common neural substrates for the addictive properties of nicotine and cocaine,' *Science* 275 (5296): pp.83–86.

20. Grant, B.F., Dawson, D.A. (1998) 'Age at onset of drug use and its association with DSM–IV drug abuse and dependence: Results from the National Longitudinal Alcohol Epidemiologic Survey,' *Journal of Substance Abuse* 10: pp.163–73.

21. Steiner, R. (1922/1976) *Lectures to the Workmen in Dornach,* Steiner Verlag, Dornach, Switzerland.

22. WHO Global Status (2004), *Report on Alcohol.*

23. Rehm, J. *et al.* (2003) 'Alcohol-related morbidity and mortality,' *Alcohol Research and Health,* 27 (1): pp.39-51.

24. Parry, C., Morojele, N., Jernigan, D. (2002) *Action for a Sober South Africa,* Alcohol & Drug Abuse Research Unit, South African Medical Research Council.

25. American Medical Association: *www.ama-assn.org/ama/pub/physician-resources/public-health/promoting-healthy-lifestyles/alcohol-other-drug-abuse.*

26. Dunn, M.E., Goldman, M.S. (1998) 'Age and drinking-related differences in the memory organization of alcohol expectancies in 3rd,

6th, 9th, and 12th grade children,' *Journal of Consulting and Clinical Psychology,* 66: pp.579–85.

27. *Quick Stats: Binge Drinking,* (April 2008) Centers for Disease Control and Prevention.

28. Stolle, M., Sack, P.M., Thomasius, R. (May 2009) 'Binge drinking in childhood and adolescence: epidemiology, consequences, and interventions,' *Dtsch Arztebl Int* 106 (19): pp.323–28.

29. Spear, L.P. (2000) 'The adolescent brain and age-related behavioral manifestations,' *Neuroscience and Biobehavioral Reviews,* 24: pp.417–63; Spear, L.P. & Varlinskaya, E.I. 'Adolescence: Alcohol sensitivity, tolerance, and intake.' In: Galanter, M., ed. (2005) *Recent Developments in Alcoholism,* Vol. 17: *Alcohol Problems in Adolescents and Young Adults: Epidemiology, Neurobiology, Prevention, Treatment,* Springer, NY, pp.143–59.

30. Clark, D.B., Lynch, K.G., Donovan, J.E., Block, G.D. (2001) 'Health problems in adolescents with alcohol use disorders: Self-report, liver injury, and physical examination findings and correlates,' *Clinical and Experimental Research,* 25: pp.1350–59.

31. Strauss, R.S., Barlow, S.E., Dietz, W.H. (2000) 'Prevalence of abnormal serum aminotransferase values in overweight and obese adolescents,' *Journal of Pediatrics,* 136: pp.727–33.

32. Mauras, N., Rogol, A.D., Haymond, M.W. & Veldhuis, J.D. (1996) 'Sex steroids, growth hormone, insulin-like growth factor-1: Neuroendocrine and metabolic regulation in puberty,' *Hormone Research,* 45:74–80.

33. Miller, D., (15-Jun-2009) 'College drinking problems, deaths on the rise,' *Journal of Studies on Alcohol and Drugs.*

34. Parliamentary Office of Science and Technology (July 2005) *Binge Drinking and Public Health,* Number 244.

35. Broughton & Walter (February 2007) *Trends in Fatal Car Accidents: Analyses of data,* Transport Research Laboratory.

36. Rosemary, T. (2006) *Most at risk are young males between 17 and 25 years,* Royal Society for the Prevention of Accidents Conference Proceedings.

37. Miller, N.S., Mahler, J.C., Gold, M.S. (1991) 'Suicide risk associated with drug and alcohol dependence,' *Journal of Addictive Diseases,* 10 (3): pp.49–61.

38. Crowell, N.A., Burgess, A.W. eds. (1996) *Understanding violence against women,* Washington DC, National Academy Press.

39. British Medical Association (2002) 'Alcohol and Young People,' *Health (2) Prevention Alert,* Vol.5, No.6, May 10.

40. Heung, C., LeMar, J., Rempel, B. (2011) 'Alcohol and Community-Based Violence: A Review of Evidence and Control Policies,' *McMaster University Medical Journal,* Volume 8 No. 1.

41. Murdoch, D., Pihl, R.O., Ross, D. (1990) 'Alcohol and crimes of violence: Present issues,' *Int J Addict,* 25: 1065-81.

42. Steiner, R. (23 May 1908/1973) *Lectures on The Gospel of St John,* Anthroposophic Press, Spring Valley, New York

43. Dunselman, R. (1995) *In Place of the Self: How Drugs Work,* Hawthorn Press, Stroud, UK.

44. Russell, M. (1990) 'Prevalence of alcoholism among children of alcoholics.' In: Windle, M., Searles, J.S., eds. *Children of Alcoholics: Critical Perspectives,* Guilford, New York, pp. 9–38.

45. Castillo Mezzich, A., Giancola, P.R., Lu, S.Y., *et al.* (1999) 'Adolescent females with a substance use disorder: Affiliations with adult male sexual partners,' *American Journal of Addictions,* 8: pp.190–200.

46. Smith, G.T., Goldman, M.S., Greenbaum, P.E., Christiansen, B.A. (1995) 'Expectancy for social facilitation from drinking: The divergent paths of high-expectancy and low-expectancy adolescents,' *Journal of Abnormal Psychology,* 104: pp.32–40.

47. Austin, E.W., Knaus, C. (2000) 'Predicting the potential for risky behavior among those 'too young' to drink as the result of appealing advertising,' *Journal of Health Communications,* 5: pp.13–27.

48. Reich, T., Edenberg, H.J., Goate, A. *et al.* (1998) 'Genome-wide search for genes affecting the risk for alcohol dependence,' *American Journal of Medical Genetics,* 81: pp.207–215. Long, J.C., Knowler, W.C., Hanson, R.L. *et al.* (1998) 'Evidence for genetic linkage to alcohol dependence on chromosomes 4 and 11 from an autosome-wide scan in an American Indian population,' *American Journal of Medical Genetics. Part B: Neuropsychiatric Genetics,* 81: pp.216–21. Foroud, T., Edenberg, H.J., Goate, A. *et al.* (2000) 'Alcoholism susceptibility loci: Confirmation studies in a replicate sample and further mapping,' *Alcoholism: Clinical and Experimental Research,* 24: pp.933–45.

49. Bauer, L.O., Hesselbrock, V.M. (1999) 'P300 decrements in teenagers with conduct problems: Implications for substance abuse risk and brain development,' *Biological Psychiatry,* 46: pp.263–72; also Bauer, L.O., and Hesselbrock, V.M. (1999) 'Subtypes of family history and conduct disorder: Effects on P300 during the Stroop Test,' *Neuropsychopharmacology,* 21: pp.51–62.

50. Tapert, S.F., Schweinsburg, A.D. (2005) 'The human adolescent brain and alcohol use disorders.' In: Galanter, M., ed. *Recent Developments in Alcoholism,* Vol. 17: *Alcohol Problems in Adolescents and Young Adults: Epidemiology, Neurobiology, Prevention, Treatment,*

Springer, New York, pp.177–97; Begleiter, H.; Porjesz, B.; Bihari, B. & Kissin, B. (1984) 'Event-related brain potentials in boys at risk for alcoholism,' *Science*, 255: pp.1493–96.

51. Goldberg, R. (2010) *Awakening to Child Health Part I* (second edition), Hawthorn Press, Stroud, UK.

52. Goldberg, R. (2007) 'Addictive Behaviour in Children, Part 2: Food and Sanctioned Substance Abuse,' *South African Journal of Natural Medicine*, Issue 29.

CHAPTER 6

1. Steiner, R. (1904/1971) *Theosophy: an introduction to the supersensible knowledge of the world and the destination of the human being*, Anthroposophic Press, New York.

2. Steiner, R. (1921/1978) 'Knowledge of Man and the Form of the Lesson,' June 13 lecture, Bibliography (GA) 302, Rudolf Steiner Press.

3. Goldberg, R. (2010) *Awakening to Child Health Part I* (second edition), Hawthorn Press, Stroud, UK.

4. This methodology integrates many years of experience as an integrative medical practitioner, Waldorf School doctor, counsellor, decades of study and clinical application in the fields of Anthroposophical Medicine, Functional Medicine and Homeopathy. This experience combined with the foundational techniques drawn from Psychophonetics Counselling, Goetheanistic science, drama and movement, arts and crafts, mythology, pedagogical medicine and other modalities, has evolved into a methodology which the author calls *Awakening to Deep Experience*. This methodology is described in publications and seminars.

5. Kaplan & Sadock's *Synopsis of Psychiatry*, eighth Edition (1998) Lippencott, Williams & Wilkins, Baltimore, Maryland USA.

6. Outram, S.M. (2010) 'The use of methylphenidate among students: the future of enhancement?' *J. Med. Ethics*, 36 (4): pp.198-20.

7. Dunselman, R. (1995) *In Place of the Self: How Drugs Work*, Hawthorn Press, Stroud UK.

8. Vogt, F. (2002) *Addiction's Many Faces*, Hawthorn Press, Stroud, UK.

9. *Awakening to Child Health Part 3 – Contemporary Therapeutic approaches to Health Disturbances in Childhood and Adolescence.* Book in progress.

CHAPTER 7

1. Patzlaff, R. (1988) *Medienmagie und die Herrschaft ueber die Sinne (Magic of the Media, Tyranny over the Senses)*, Verlag Freies Geistesleben, Stuttgart.

2. Postman, N. (1994) *The Disappearance of Childhood*, Vintage Books, New York.

3. McDonough, P. (October 26, 2009) *TV viewing among kids at an eight-year high:* http://blog.nielsen.com/nielsenwire/media.

4. Rideout, V.J., Vandewater, E.A., Wartella, E.A. (2003) *Zero to six: electronic media in the lives of infants, toddlers and preschoolers*, Kaiser Family Foundation, Menlo Park CA.

5. Rideout, V.J., Foehr, U.G., Roberts, D.F. (January 2010) *Media in the lives of 8-18 year-olds*, Kaiser Family Foundation.

6. Gigli, S., (April 2004) *Children,Youth and Media Around the World: An Overview of Trends & Issues*, Inter Media Survey Institute, for UNICEF.

7. Postman, N. (1993) *Technopoly The Surrender of Culture to Technology*, Vintage Books, New York.

8. Thakkar, R.R., Garrison, M.M., Christakis, D.A. (2006) 'A systematic review for the effects of television viewing by infants and preschoolers,' *Pediatrics*, 118: pp.2025–2031.

9. *Children, adolescents and television* (2001) American Academy of Pediatrics, Committee on Public Education, *Pediatrics*, 107 (2): pp.423–426.

10. Christakis, D.A., Zimmerman, F.J., DiGiuseppe, D.L., McCarty, C.A. (2004) 'Early television exposure and subsequent attentional problems in children,' *Pediatrics*, 113 (4): pp.708-713.

11. Zimmerman, F.J., Christakis, D.A. (2005 July) 'Children's television viewing and cognitive outcomes: a longitudinal analysis of national data,' *Arch Pediatr Adolesc Med*, 159 (7): pp.619–25.

12. Large, M. (29 Sept 2006) *Toxic TV: How the TV Medium affects children's learning:* Martinhclarge@gmail.com.

13. Healy, J. (1991) *Endangered Minds. Why children don't think and what we can do about it*, Touchstone Books.

14. Healy, J. (1994) *Your Child's Growing Mind: A Guide to Learning and Brain Development from Birth to Adolescence*, Doubleday.

15. Noel, J. (July 2003) 'Effects of Media on Early Brain Development,' research Paper, *Electronic Media*.

16. Hancox, R.J., Milne, B.J., Poulton, R. (2005 July) 'Association of television viewing during childhood with poor educational achievement,' *Arch Pediatr Adolesc Med*, 159 (7): pp.614–18.

17. Lumeng, J.C., Rahnama, S., Appugliese, D., Kaciroti, N., Bradley, R.H. (2006 April) 'Television exposure and overweight risk in pre-schoolers,' *Arch Pediatr Adolesc Med*, 160 (4): pp.417–22.

18. Viner, R.M., Cole, T.J. (2005) 'Television viewing in early childhood predicts adult body mass index,' *J Pediatr*, Oct. 147 (4): pp.429–35.

19. Jago, R., Baranowski, T., Baranowski, J.C., Thompson D., Greaves K.A. (2005 June) 'BMI from 3–6 years of age is predicted by TV viewing and physical activity, not diet,' *Int J Obes*, (Lond) 29 (6): pp.557–64.

20. Klesges, R.C., Shelton, M.L., Klesges, L.M. (1993 Feb) 'Effects of television on metabolic rate: potential implications for childhood obesity,' *Pediatrics*, 91(2):281-6.

21. Mok, T.A. (1998) 'Getting the message: media images and stereotypes and their effect on Asian Americans,' *Cult Divers Ment Health*, 4 (3): pp.185–202.

22. Coltrane, S., Messineo, M. (2000 Mar) 'The perpetuation of subtle prejudice: race and gender imagery in 1990s television advertising,' *Sex Roles*, 42 (5/6): pp.363–89.

23. Tamburro, R.F., Gordon, P.L, D'Apolito, J.P., Howard, S.C. (2004 Dec) 'Unsafe and violent behavior in commercials aired during tel-evised major sporting events,' *Pediatrics*, 114 (6): pp.694–8.

26. American Academy of Pediatrics, Committee on Public Education. (2001) 'Media violence,' *Pediatrics*, Nov. 108 (5): pp.1222-26.

25. Williams, C.L. *et al.* (2002) 'Cardiovascular Health in Childhood,' *Circulation*, 106: pp.143–60.

26. Bushman, B.J., Anderson, C.A. (2009) 'Comfortably numb: desensi-tizing effects of violent media on helping others,' *Psychological Science*, 21 (3): pp.273–77.

27. Steiner, R. (9.10.1918) *The Work of the Angels in Man's Astral Body*, Lecture in Zurich.

28. Postman, N. (1986) *Amusing Ourselves to Death*, Heinemann, London.

CHAPTER 8

1. Kaiser Family Foundation (2003) *Zero to Six: Media Use in the Lives of Infants, Toddlers, and Preschoolers*, Kaiser Family Foundation, Menlo Park, CA.

2. Kaiser Family Foundation (2005) *Generation M: Media in the Lives of 8–18 Year Olds*, Kaiser Family Foundation, Menlo Park, CA.

3. Anderson, D.R., & Evans, M.K. (2001) 'Peril and Potential of Media for Infants and Toddlers,' *Zero to Three*, October/November, 22 (2), pp.11, 14.

4. Carnes, P.J., Murray, R.E., Carpentier, L., (2005) 'Bargains With Chaos: Sex Addicts and Addiction Interaction Disorder,' *Sexual Addiction & Compulsivity*, 12: pp.79–120.

5. Emberson, P. (1997) *The Internet and the World Wide Web*, New View Journal.

6. King, P. *The Incarnation of Ahriman* (unpublished article).

7. White, R. (2006) *How Computers Work*, eighth edition, Que Publishing, Indianapolis.

8. *Fool's Gold: A Critical Look at Computers in Children.* (2001) Edited by Colleen Cordes & Edward Miller, Alliance for Childhood.

9. Valdemar,W., Setzer, V.W., Duckett, G.E. (1992) *The Risks to Children using Electronic Games*, Proceedings Vol. 2, p.471.

10. Pascarelli, E., Quilter, D. (1994) *Repetitive Strain Injury: A Computer User's Guide*, Wiley Publishers, NY.

11. Armstrong, A., Casement, C. (May 2000) *The Child and the Machine: How Computers Put Our Children's Education at Risk*, Gryphon House Publishers.

12. Martin, James A. (2000-06-09) 'The Pain of Portable Computing,' *PC World*, retrieved 2008-11-27.

13. Mooney, L. (Oct 8, 2009) *Computer Vision Syndrome:* http://www.livestrong.com/article/25560-computer-vision-syndrome/#ixzz1a5a0fIts.

14. Palmer, S. (1993) 'Does computer use put children's vision at risk?' *Journal of Research and Development in Education*, Vol. 26, No. 2, pp.59–65.

15. Palmer, S. (1984) 'Transient Myopia after Visual Work,' *Ergonomics*, Vol.2, No.11.

16. Vitale, S., Sperduto,R.D., Ferris, F.L., (December 2009) *Increased prevalence of myopia in the United States between 1971-1972 and 1999-2004*, Archives of Ophthalmology.

17. Lobstein, T., Baur, L, Uauy, R., (2004) 'Obesity in children and young people: a crisis in public health,' *Obes Rev 5*, supplement 1: pp.4–85.

18. Wang, Y., Lobstein, T., (2006) 'Worldwide trends in childhood overweight and obesity,' *International Journal of Pediatric Obesity*, Vol.1: No.1, pp.11–25.

19. Ogden, C.L., Carroll, M.D., Flegal, K.M. (May 2008) 'High body mass index for age among US children and adolescents,' *JAMA* 299 (20): pp.2401–5: doi:10.1001/jama.299.20.2401, PMID 18505949.

20. Steinberger, J., Moran, A., Hong, C.P., Jacobs, D.R. Jr, Sinaiko, A.R. (2001) 'Adiposity in childhood predicts obesity and insulin resistance in young adulthood,' *J Pediatr*, 138: pp.469–473.

21. Healey, J. M. (1998) *Failure to Connect: How Computers affect our children's minds – for better and worse*, Simon & Schuster, NY.

22. Hampton, K., Sessions, L., Her, E.J. (Nov 2009)'How the Internet and mobile phones impact American's social network,' *Social Isolation and New Technology.*

23. Gross, E.F. (2004) 'Adolescent Internet use: What we expect, what teens report,' *Applied Developmental Psychology,* 25: pp.633–49.

24. Sloan, D. (1985) *The Computer in Education: A Critical perspective,* Teachers College Press, NY.

25. Sanders, B. (1994) *A is for Ox: Violence, Electronic Media and the Silencing of the Written Word,* Pantheon, NY.

26. Healy, J.M. (1998) *Failure to Connect: How Computers Affect Our Children's Minds – for better and worse,* Simon & Schuster, NY.

27. Dworak, M., Schierl, T., Bruns, T., Strueder, H.K. (2007) 'Impact of Singular Excessive Computer Game and Television Exposure on Sleep Patterns and Memory Performance of School-aged Children,' *Pediatrics,* November 1, Vol.120, No.5, pp.978–85.

CHAPTER 9

1. Omar, S., Wild, A. (2005) *Research into the Dynamics of Young Sex Offenders in Venda,* Research conducted for Thouyandou Victim Empowerment Trust.

2. Shaw, D., Fernandes, J.R., Chitra, R., (December 2005) 'Suicide in Children and Adolescents: A 10-Year Retrospective Review,' *American Journal of Forensic Medicine & Pathology,* Vol.26, 4, pp.309–15.

3. Centers for Disease Control and Prevention, (Dec 2007) 'Trends Among Youths and Young Adults aged 10–24,' *Morbidity and Mortality Weekly Report,* 56 (35), pp.905–8.

4. Gloeckler, M. & Goebel, W. (2003) *A Guide to Child Health,* Floris Books, Edinburgh.

5. Goldberg. R. (2010) *Awakening to Child Health Part I* (second edition), Hawthorn Press, Stroud, UK.

6. Lievegoed, B. (1985) *Phases of Childhood,* Floris Books, Edinburgh, UK.

7. Tagar, Y. Internal training material of Persephone Institute of Psychophonetics.

8. Kaplan & Sadock, eds. (1998) *Synopsis of Psychiatry,* eighth edition, Lippencott, Williams & Wilkins Baltimore, Maryland USA.

9. Field, E.M. (2007) *Bullying Blocking,* Finch Publishing, Sydney, Australia.

10. Kowalski, R.M., Limber, S.P., Agatston, P.W. (2008) *Cyber Bullying: Bullying in the Digital Age,* Blackwell, Oxford.

11. David-Ferdon, C., Hertz, M.F., (2007) 'Electronic media, violence,

and adolescents: an emerging public health problem,' *Journal of Adolescent Health*, 41 (supplement 1): pp.S1–S5.

12. Wolak, J., Mitchell, K.J., Finkelhor, D. (2007) 'Does online harassment constitute bullying? An exploration of online harassment by known peers and online-only contacts,' *Journal of Adolescent Health*, 41 (supplement 1): pp.S51–58.

13. McVey-Nobel, M., Khenlani-Patel, S., Neziroglu, F. (2006) *When your child is cutting. A parent's guide to helping children overcome self-injury*, New Harbinger Publications, Oakland CA.

14. Favazza, A. (1998) 'The coming of age of self-mutilation,' *Journal of Nervous and Mental Disease*, 186 (5): pp.259–68.

15. DiClement, R. *et al.* (1991) 'Prevalence and correlates of cutting behaviour,' *Journal of the American Academy of Child and Adolescent Psychiatry*, 30 (5): pp.735–39.

16. Herpertz, S, Sass, H., Favazza, A.R. (1997) 'Impulsivity in self-mutilative behaviour: Psychometric and biological findings,' *Journal of Psychiatric Research*, 31 (4): pp.451–65.

17. Winchel, R., Stanley, M. (1991) 'Self-injurious behaviour: A review of the behaviour and biology of self-mutilation,' *American Journal of Psychiatry*, 148: pp.306–17.

18. Pelkonen, M., Martunen, M. (2003) 'Child and adolescent suicide: epidemiology, risk factors, and approaches to prevention,' *Paediat Drugs*,5 (4): pp.243–65.

19. Tagar, Y., Goldberg, R. 'Transforming the Enemy: A Psycho-spiritual-somatic Approach to Auto-Immune Disorders using Medical Psychophonetics. A Foundation Paper for Participatory Medicine.' (Unpublished article)

20. Sachsse, U., Von Der Heyde, S., G. Huether (2002) 'Stress regulation and self-mutilation,' *Americal Journal of Psychiatry*, 159(4): p.672.

21. Greydanus, D.E., Pratt, H.D., Spates, Richard C., Blake-Dreher, A.E., Greydanus-Gearhart, M.A., Patel, D.R. (May 2003). 'Corporal punishment in schools: position paper of the Society for Adolescent Medicine,' *Journal of Adolescent Health*, 32 (5): pp.385–93.

22. Palmer, Sue (2007) *Toxic Childhood*, Orion Books, London.

23. Fitzgerald, Randall (2006) *The Hundred Year Lie How Food And Medicine Are Destroying Your Health*, Dutton Adult, USA.

24. World Health Organization (2002*) World Report on Violence and Health. Drugs, Alcohol and Violence*, Geneva; Lauer, Hans E. (1981) *Aggression and Repression*, Rudolf Steiner Press, London.

25. Goldberg, R. (2002) 'Mommy, where do I come from?' *South African Journal of Natural Medicine*, Issue 8.

26. American Academy of Pediatrics, Committee on Public Education. (2001) 'Media violence,' *Pediatrics,* Nov. 108 (5): pp.1222-26.

27. Senate Judiciary Committee Media Violence Report: (1999) *Children, Violence and the Media.*

28. Huesmann, L.R. (1986) 'Psychological processes promoting the relation between exposure to media violence and aggressive behaviour by the viewer,' *Journal of Social Issues,* 42: pp.125–39.

29. Huesmann, L.R., & L.D. Eron (1986) *Television and the Aggressive Child: A Cross-National Comparison,* Lawrence Erlbaum Associates, Hillsdale, NJ.

30. Grossman, Dave (1996) *On Killing: The Psychological Cost of Learning to Kill in War and Society,* Little Brown & Co., Boston, New York, London.

31. Goldberg, R. (2004) *The Challenge of Stress in Childhood: Awaken to Child Health No.13,* Dreamcatcher Publications.

32. Goldberg, R. (2004) *Communicating With Stressed Children: Awaken to Child Health No.1,* Dreamcatcher Publications.

CHAPTER 10

1. *Cape Times* front page headlines: October 23, 2006.

2. Omar, Shaheda (2006) *Research into the Dynamics of Young Sex offenders in Venda.* Research conducted for Thoyandou Victim Empowerment Trust.

3. Schewe, P.A. (2006) *Interventions to prevent sexual violence.* In L.S. Doll, S.E. Bonzo, J.A. Mercy, D.A. Sleet, *eds. Handbook of Injury and Violence Prevention,* pp.223–40, Springer, New York.

4. Kilpatrick, D.G., Edmunds, C.N., Seymour, A.K. (1992) *Rape in America: A report to the nation,* Arlington, TX: National Victim Center and Medical University of South Carolina.

5. Loh, C., Gidycz, C.A., Lobo, T.R., Luthra, R. (2005) 'A prospective analysis of sexual assault perpetration: Risk factors related to perpetrator characteristics,' *Journal of Interpersonal Violence,* 20, pp.1325–48.

6. World Health Organization (2001) *World Report on Violence and Health,* Geneva, Switzerland.

7. Shaw, J. (2000) 'Child on child sexual abuse: Psychological perspectives,' *Child Abuse & Neglect,* 24 (12): pp.1591–1600.

8. Grant, J., Indermaur, D., Thornton, J., Stevens, G., Chamarette, C., & Halse, A. (2009) *Intrafamilial adolescent sex offenders: psychological profile and treatment,* Trends and Issues in Crime and Criminal Justice No. 375.

9. Goldberg, R. (2010) *Awakening to Child Health Part I* (second edition), Hawthorn Press, Stroud, UK.

10. Groth, N. (1979) *Men Who Rape: The Psychology of the Offender,* Plenum Press, New York, pp.44–45.

11. Dean, K.E., Malamuth, N.M. (1997) 'Characteristics of men who aggress sexually and of men who imagine aggressing: risk and moderating variables,' *Journal of Personality and Social Psychology,* 72: pp.449–55.

12. Walters, P.A., (March 2010) 'Promiscuity in Adolescence,' *American Journal of Orthopsychiatry.*

13. American Academy of Child and Adolescent Psychiatry Committee On Public Education (January 2001) 'Sexuality, Contraception and the Media,' *Pediatrics,* 107 (1): pp.191–99.

14. Willis, B.M., Levy, B.S., (2002) 'Child prostitution: global health burden, research needs, and interventions,' *The Lancet,* V359 (9315), pp.1417–22; Meier, E. (2002) 'Child Rape in South Africa,' *Pediatric Nursing,* 28 (5).

15. Lievegoed, B. (1985) *Phases of Childhood,* Floris Books, Edinburgh, UK.

16. Gaedeke, W. (1998) *Sexuality, Partnership and Marriage,* Temple Lodge, London.

17. Louw, D.A., Van Ede, D.M., Loue, A.E (1998) *Human Development* (second ed.), Kagiso Publishers, Pretoria.

18. Du Toit, B.M. (1987) 'Menarche and sexuality among a sample of black South African schoolgirls,' *Social Sciences and Medicine,* 24, pp.501–71.

19. Goldberg, R. (2004) *Communicating With Stressed Children, Awaken to Child Health No.1,* Dreamcatcher Publications.

20. Steiner, R. (9.10.1918) 'The Work of the Angels in Man's Astral Body,' Lecture in Zurich.

CHAPTER 11

1. Steiner, R. (1999) *A Psychology of Body, Soul and Spirit,* 4 lectures, Nov 1–4, 1910 Anthroposophic Press, Hudson, NY.

2. Tagar, Y. (1986–2006) *Psychophonetics. A Collection of Articles,* Persephone Institute for Psychophonetics.

3. Steele, R. (2005) 'A hermeneutic phenomenological study of/in transformation: An embodied and creative exploration of therapeutic change through Psychophonetics psychotherapy.' Doctoral dissertation. Edith Cowan University, Western Australia.

4. Steele, R. (2011) *Psychophonetics: Holistic Counseling and Psychotherapy: Stories and Insights from Practice,* Lindisfarne Books, NY.

5. Goldberg, R. (2010) *Awakening to Child Health: Part 1* (second ed.), Hawthorn Press, Stroud, Chapter 6.

CHAPTER 12

1. Goldberg, R. (2010) *Awakening to Child Health: Part 1* (second ed.), Hawthorn Press, Stroud, Chapter 7.
2. Goldberg, R. (2010) Chapter 8.
3. Goldberg, R. (2010) Chapter 9.

APPENDIX 1: A Blueprint for Understanding and Managing Addictions in Childhood and Young Adults

1. A willingness to help

2. Understanding the nature of addiction: Chapter 2, p. 36–39.
   - needs and gratification: Chapter 1, p. 18–22.
   - dependency: Chapter 2, p. 23.
   - road map of holistic child and adolescent development: Chapter 2, p. 30–36.
   - psychodynamics of addiction: Chapter 2, p. 38f
   - environment of addiction: Chapter 2, p. 40f.

3. Check yourself and care for yourself: Chapters 2, 3, p. 27–29, p. 47

4. Understand the specific child in your care and his or her needs: Chapter 3, p. 47–50.
   - developmental phase of the child, p. 32–36
   - child's constitution, temperament, character, p. 235f
   - perspective of the child's environment, p. 40f

5. Detect the warning signs of addiction: Chapters 4-10

6. Assess the degree of your child's addictive behaviour: Chapters 4–10
   - accurate picture; state of health; extent; frequency; duration: Chapter 3, p. 49f

7. Awaken deep insight: Chapters 2, 3, Appendix 2
   - observe child profile (physical/sensory-kinaesthetic-auditory-tonal-thought-ego profile): p. 28;
   - imitate the child consciously and empathetically through gesture or role play: p. 28f

- observe own gesture and imitation and discover new picture-meaning;
- explore compassionate understanding/attitudinal change: p. 49;
- determine your new meeting and your new position with regard to the child.

8. Principal insights
   - behind all addictive behaviour there hides a vulnerable and needy child whose inner soul needs have not been addressed and who will need outer support and inner skills to empower him or herself;
   - the environment needs to change where possible from a negative, toxic and destructive one into a positive, healthy and supportive one;
   - the child needs guidance to understand his or her issues and to acquire the inner skills and resources to help him or herself.

9. Foundational management: Chapters 4–11
   - establish effective communication;
   - show interest and respect – learn to listen;
   - create a partnership and teamwork;
   - establish your own ethical guidelines;
   - create motivation, commitment, contracts, accountability and realistic time frames.

10. Clinical management
    - individual dietary and nutritional interventions;
    - detox programmes using oral and intravenous procedures;
    - individually prescribed neutraceutical, herbal and homeopathic medication;
    - a range of therapeutic options such as rhythmical massage, art therapy, movement therapy;
    - age-specific counselling;
    - referral to specialist care and rehab centres.

APPENDIX 2: Awakening to Deep Experience – Learning to experience the nature of addiction with artistic representation of some addictive agencies

In normal waking consciousness, we experience the world in only four ways: through our cognitive functions of thinking, remembering and visualising, our sensing and perceiving functions, our feeling or emotive responses, and our expressive, intuitive and will based actions. All interactions and all learning take place through the four psychological activities.

When we become conscious of these four basic functions of experience, we can sharpen and strengthen these capacities and through constant practice become a knower of life. We can thereby become a real expert in any field of life. We can also turn the spotlight on ourselves and discover who we really are. We begin to recognise the vast potential that lies hidden within, and we may start to make use of it for our benefit and fulfilment, as well as for the good of others.

These natural capacities of the human psyche can thus become self- empowering tools that can be taught to all who seek to deepen their experience of life and wish to empower themselves to become active carers of both themselves and the world.

This book on addictive behaviour was written by applying these self-empowering tools to the subject of addiction; it was also written with the conviction that anyone who applies themselves consciously and diligently to developing these skills, can arrive at a deep knowing experience of the addictive phenomenon. The book offers a tried and tested method to understand and effectively support young people caught up in addictive behaviour. This approach is outlined in Chapters 2, 3 and Appendix 1, and in the following chapters is applied to the specific addictions with case histories and management guidelines.

This approach which is summarised in Appendix 1, will be enhanced through strengthening the four basic functions of human experience, and the more skilled we are in using them, the more we will be able to understand and care for the addicted youth. We will examine the various steps and see which psychological activity can be strengthened for maximum efficacy:

1. The willingness to help the child challenges our motivation, intention and resolves: for this we need to strengthen our *will* forces.

2. Understanding the nature of addiction, needs and gratification, dependency, the road map of holistic child and adolescent development, and the psychodynamics of addiction, primarily calls on developing clear unprejudiced *thinking*, but also on enhancing deep curiosity and interest to know (*will* activity), strengthening imagination (a kind of internal *seeing*) and developing heart empathy (*insightful and compassionate feelings*).

3. Checking and caring for yourself requires developing the skill of self-reflection, strengthening those functions of internal *sensing* and *feeling*, the *will* to step aside, seeing oneself and discovering a new kind of imaginative *thinking* which can give new meaning to new perceptions of self.

4. Understanding the specific child in your care, his needs, his developmental phase, his constitution, temperament, character and environment.

5. Detecting the warning signs of addiction: will call on enhancing the same activities as point 2. It will also require deepening the art of *sensing*.

6. Assessing the degree of your child's addictive behaviour: will challenge the same activities as point 5.

7. Awakening to deep insight will call on utilising and enhancing the full spectrum of *sensing*: the sense of balance and movement, of touch, sight, hearing and smell, and the finer sense for tone, the thought life of the child and the sense of his unique individuality. Conscious imitation will require the *will* to enter and to dramatically express the child's inner nature, as well as deep empathy (feeling/willing) and unprejudiced *thinking*. New meetings and new positions will call on motivation, intention, resolve and action, which are all aspects of strengthening the life of will.

8. Principal insights call on developing a kind of *thinking* that can capture the essence of things.
9. Foundational and clinical management and call on the heightened ability to put into action all the insights gained above (*will*).

Many of the indications given in this book for helping children and youth trapped in addictive behaviour are based on common sense and can immediately be applied by the reader to their own personal encounters with children in their care. Other indications however will generally require further instruction or training for them to be properly implemented. For instance the dramatic characterisation of the dependent child or the addictive agency will require guidance and coaching of the kind that takes place in personal counselling sessions or workshops.

Through the experiences gained in hundreds of sessions working with addictions of many kinds, it was possible, working with an intuitive artist, to create an artistic representation of some of the addictive agencies. The pictures illustrated below may give some an artistic experience of what is described in the book. These pictures are, I believe, a true characterisation of at least some aspects of these agencies.

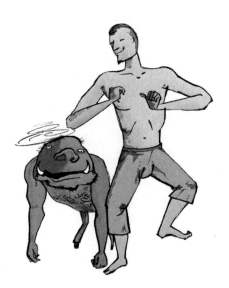

Alcohol addiction

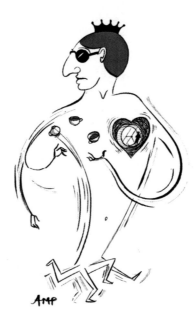

Caffeine addiction

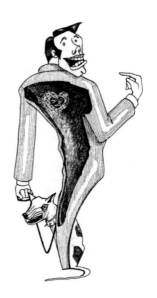

Cocaine addiction

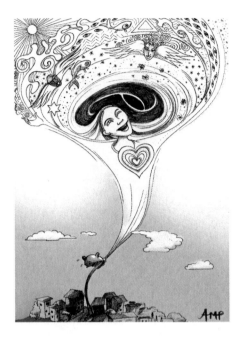

Cosmic addiction

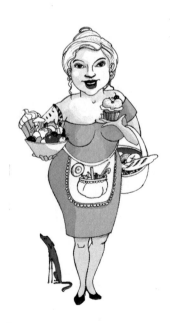

Food addiction

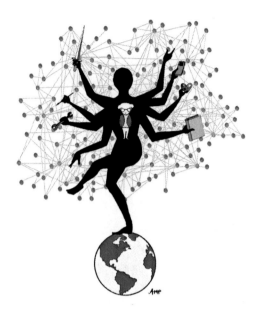

Internet addiction

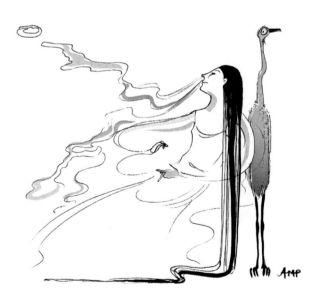

Nicotine addiction

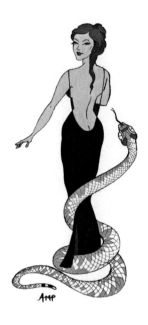

Sex addiction

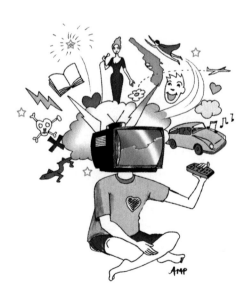

TV addiction

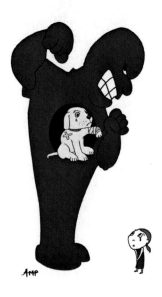

Violence addiction

There may be some readers who would wish to enter more deeply into the experience of addiction, and would wish to apply this methodology in the pursuit of gaining deeper insight in the manner described above. In this regard, this book was not intended as an instruction manual for self-exploration, but rather as an indicator of possibilities and a referral point for a professionally guided coaching or training. Readers are referred to the following websites for personal instruction through counselling coaching sessions, seminars or training courses:

www.drraoulgoldberg.com
www.syringahealth.co.za.
www.psychophonetics.com

Bibliography

American Academy of Child and Adolescent Psychiatry, Committee on Public Education (January 2001) 'Sexuality, Contraception and the Media,' *Pediatrics,* 107 (1): pp.191–99.

American Academy of Pediatrics, Committee on Public Education (2001) 'Children, adolescents and television,' *Pediatrics,* 107 (2): pp.423–26.

American Academy of Pediatrics, Committee on Public Education (2001) 'Media violence,' *Pediatrics,* Nov. 108 (5): pp.1222-26.

American Medical Association: *www.ama-assn.org/ama/pub/physician-resources/public-health/promoting-healthy-lifestyles/alcohol-other-drug-abuse.*

Anderson, D.R., & Evans, M.K. (2001) 'Peril and Potential of Media for Infants and Toddlers,' *Zero to Three,* October/November, 22 (2), pp.11, 14.

Arias-Carrión, O., Pöppel, E. (2007) 'Dopamine, learning, reward-seeking behaviour,' *Act Neurobiol Exp,* 67 (4): pp.481–88.

Armstrong, A., Casement, C. (May 2000) *The Child and the Machine: How Computers Put Our Children's Education at Risk,* Gryphon House Publishers.

Austin, E.W., Knaus, C. (2000) 'Predicting the potential for risky behavior among those 'too young' to drink as the result of appealing advertising,' *Journal of Health Communications,* 5: pp.13–27.

Barone, J.J., Roberts, H.R. (14 August 1995) *Caffeine Consumption,* National Soft Drink Association.

Bauer, L.O. & Hesselbrock, V.M. (1999) 'P300 decrements in teenagers with conduct problems: Implications for substance abuse risk and brain development,' *Biological Psychiatry,* 46: pp.263–72.

—, & Hesselbrock, V.M. (1999) 'Subtypes of family history and conduct disorder: Effects on P300 during the Stroop Test,' *Neuropsychopharmacology,* 21: pp.51–62.

Begleiter, H., Porjesz, B., Bihari, B. & Kissin, B. (1984) 'Event-related brain potentials in boys at risk for alcoholism,' *Science,* 255: pp.1493–96.

Bernstein, G. A., Carroll, M.E., Thuras, P.D., *et al.* (2002) 'Caffeine dependence in teenagers,' *Drug and Alcohol Dependence*, 66, pp.1–6.

British Medical Association (2002) 'Alcohol and Young People,' *Health (2) Prevention Alert*, Vol.5, No.6, May 10.

Broughton & Walter (February 2007) *Trends in Fatal Car Accidents: Analyses of data*, Transport Research Laboratory.

Bushman, B.J., Anderson, C.A. (2009) 'Comfortably numb: desensitizing effects of violent media on helping others,' *Psychological Science*, 21(3): pp.273–77.

Caffeine Content of Drinks, Energy Fiend (2011-03-04): www.energy-fiend.com/the-caffeine-database

Caffeine Content of Food and Drugs (2009-08-03) Nutrition Action Health Newsletter, Centre for Science in the Public Interest.

Cape Times front page headlines: October 23, 2006.

Carnes, P.J., Murray, R.E., Carpentier, L. (2005) 'Bargains With Chaos: Sex Addicts and Addiction Interaction Disorder,' *Sexual Addiction & Compulsivity*, 12: pp.79–120.

Castillo Mezzich, A., Giancola, P.R., Lu, S.Y., *et al.* (1999) 'Adolescent females with a substance use disorder: Affiliations with adult male sexual partners,' *American Journal of Addictions*, 8: pp.190–200.

Centers for Disease Control and Prevention (CDC) (2007) 'High School Students Who Tried to Quit Smoking Cigarettes,' *Morbidity and Mortality Weekly Report*, 58 (16): pp.428-31.

—, (CDC) (2007) 'Trends Among Youths and Young Adults aged 10–24,' *Morbidity and Mortality Weekly Report*, December, 56 (35), pp.905–8.

— (CDC) (April 2008) *Quick Stats: Binge Drinking*.

—, (CDC) (2009) 'Cigarette smoking among adults and trends in smoking cessation,' *Morbidity and Mortality Weekly Report*, 58 (44): pp.1227–32.

Charlesworth A, Glantz S.A. (2005) 'Smoking in the movies increases adolescent smoking: a review,' *Pediatrics*, Dec. 116 (6): pp.1516–28.

Chassin, L., Presson, C., Rose, J., Sherman, S.J., Prost, J. (2002) 'Parental Smoking Cessation and Adolescent Smoking,' *Journal of Pediatric Psychology*, 27 (6): pp.485–96.

Christakis, D.A., Zimmerman, F.J., DiGiuseppe, D.L., McCarty, C.A. (2004) 'Early television exposure and subsequent attentional problems in children,' *Pediatrics*, 113 (4): pp.708-713.

Clark, D.B., Lynch, K.G., Donovan, J.E., Block, G.D. (2001) 'Health problems in adolescents with alcohol use disorders: Self-report, liver injury, and physical examination findings and correlates,' *Clinical and*

Experimental Research, 25: pp.1350–59.

Coltrane, S., Messineo, M. (2000) 'The perpetuation of subtle prejudice: race and gender imagery in 1990s television advertising,' *Sex Roles,* March, 42 (5/6): pp.363–89.

Crowell, N.A., Burgess, A.W. eds. (1996) *Understanding violence against women,* Washington DC, National Academy Press.

Daly, J.W., Fredholm, B.B. (1998) 'Caffeine – an atypical drug of dependence,' *Drug and Alcohol Dependence,* 51: pp.199–206.

David-Ferdon, C., Hertz, M.F., (2007) 'Electronic media, violence, and adolescents: an emerging public health problem,' *Journal of Adolescent Health,* 41, (supplement 1): pp.S1–5.

Dean, K.E., Malamuth, N.M. (1997) 'Characteristics of men who aggress sexually and of men who imagine aggressing: risk and moderating variables,' *Journal of Personality and Social Psychology,* 72: pp.449–55.

Derenne, J.L., Beresin, E.V. (May-June 2006) 'Body Image, Media, and Eating Disorders,' *Acad Psychiatry,* 30: pp.257-61.

DiClement, R. *et al.* (1991) 'Prevalence and correlates of cutting behaviour,' *Journal of the American Academy of Child and Adolescent Psychiatry,* 30 (5): pp.735–39.

Du Toit, B.M. (1987) 'Menarche and sexuality among a sample of black South African schoolgirls,' *Social Sciences and Medicine,* 24, pp.501–71.

Dunn, M.E., Goldman, M.S. (1998) 'Age and drinking-related differences in the memory organization of alcohol expectancies in 3rd, 6th, 9th, and 12th grade children,' *Journal of Consulting and Clinical Psychology,* 66: pp.579–85.

Dunselman, R. (1995) *In Place of the Self: How Drugs Work,* Hawthorn Press, Stroud, UK.

Dworak, M., Schierl, T., Bruns, T., Strueder, H.K. (November 1, 2007) 'Impact of Singular Excessive Computer Game and Television Exposure on Sleep Patterns and Memory Performance of School-aged Children,' *Pediatrics,* Vol.120, No.5, pp.978–85.

Emberson, P. (1997) *The Internet and the World Wide Web,* New View Journal.

Favazza, A. (1998) 'The coming of age of self-mutilation,' *Journal of Nervous and Mental Disease,* 186 (5): pp.259–68.

Feltenstein, M.W. (2008 May) 'The neurocircuitry of addiction: an overview,' *British Journal of Pharmacology,* 154 (2): pp.261–74.

Field, E.M. (2007) *Bullying Blocking,* Finch Publishing, Sidney, Australia.

Fitzgerald, Randall (2006) *The Hundred Year Lie How Food And Medicine Are Destroying Your Health,* Dutton Adult, USA.

Foroud, T., Edenberg, H.J., Goate, A. *et al.* (2000) 'Alcoholism susceptibility loci: Confirmation studies in a replicate sample and further mapping,' *Alcoholism: Clinical and Experimental Research,* 24: pp.933–45.

Fool's Gold: A Critical Look at Computers in Children (2001) Edited by Colleen Cordes & Edward Miller, Alliance for Childhood.

Gaedeke, W. (1998) *Sexuality, Partnership and Marriage,* Temple Lodge, London.

Gloeckler, M. & Goebel, W. (2003) *A Guide to Child Health,* Floris Books, Edinburgh.

Goldberg, R. (2002) 'Mommy, where do I come from?' *South African Journal of Natural Medicine,* Issue 8.

—, (2004) *Communicating With Stressed Children: Awaken to Child Health No.1,* Dreamcatcher Publications.

—, (2004) *The Challenge of Stress in Childhood: Awaken to Child Health No.13,* Dreamcatcher Publications.

—, (2006) 'Eating Disorders in Children,' *Natural Medicine,* Issue 23.

—, (2007) 'Addictive Behaviour in Children, Part 2: Food and Sanctioned Substance Abuse,' *South African Journal of Natural Medicine,* Issue 29.

—, (2007–8) Articles written for *South African Journal of Natural Medicine.*

—, (2010) *Awakening to Child Health Part I* (second edition), Hawthorn Press, Stroud, UK.

—, *Awakening to Child Health Part 3 – Contemporary Therapeutic approaches to Health Disturbances in Childhood and Adolescence.* Book in progress.

—, *Awakening to Deep Experience:* www.drraoulgoldberg.com, www.syringahealth.co.za.

Grant, B.F., Dawson, D.A. (1998) 'Age at onset of drug use and its association with DSM–IV drug abuse and dependence: Results from the National Longitudinal Alcohol Epidemiologic Survey,' *Journal of Substance Abuse,* 10: pp.163–73.

Grant, J., Indermaur, D., Thornton, J., Stevens, G., Chamarette, C., & Halse, A. (2009) *Intrafamilial adolescent sex offenders: psychological profile and treatment,* Trends and Issues in Crime and Criminal Justice No.375.

Greydanus, D.E., Pratt, H.D., Spates, Richard C., Blake-Dreher, A.E., Greydanus-Gearhart, M.A., Patel, D.R. (May 2003). 'Corporal punishment in schools: position paper of the Society for Adolescent Medicine,' *Journal of Adolescent Health*, 32 (5): pp.385–93.

Gross, E.F. (2004) 'Adolescent Internet use: What we expect, what teens report,' *Applied Developmental Psychology*, 25: pp.633–49.

Grossman, Dave (1996) *On Killing: The Psychological Cost of Learning to Kill in War and Society*, Little Brown & Co., Boston, New York, London.

Groth, N. (1979) *Men Who Rape: The Psychology of the Offender*, Plenum Press, New York, pp.44–45.

Hampton, K., Sessions, L., Her, E.J. (Nov 2009)'How the Internet and mobile phones impact American's social network,' *Social Isolation and New Technology*.

Hancox, R.J., Milne, B.J., Poulton, R. (2005 July) 'Association of television viewing during childhood with poor educational achievement,' *Arch Pediatr Adolesc Med*, 159 (7): pp.614–18.

Harwood, A.C. (1967) *The Way of a Child*, Rudolf Steiner Press, London.

—, (1982) *The Recovery of Man in Childhood*, Anthroposophic Press, Spring Valley, NY.

Healy, Jane M. (1991) *Endangered Minds. Why children don't think and what we can do about it*, Touchstone Books.

—, (1994) *Your Child's Growing Mind: A Guide to Learning and Brain Development from Birth to Adolescence*, Doubleday.

—, (1998) *Failure to Connect: How computers affect our children's minds – for better and worse*, Simon & Schuster, NY.

Hering-Hanit, R. & Gadoth, N. (2003) 'Caffeine-induced headache in children and adolescents,' *Cephalalgia*, 23, pp.332–335.

Herpertz, S, Sass, H., Favazza, A.R. (1997) 'Impulsivity in self-mutilative behaviour: Psychometric and biological findings,' *Journal of Psychiatric Research*, 31 (4): pp.451–65.

Heung, C., LeMar, J., Rempel, B. (2011) 'Alcohol and Community-Based Violence: A Review of Evidence and Control Policies,' *McMaster University Medical Journal*, Volume 8 No. 1.

Huesmann, L.R. (1986) 'Psychological processes promoting the relation between exposure to media violence and aggressive behaviour by the viewer,' *Journal of Social Issues*, 42: pp.125–39.

—, & L.D. Eron (1986) *Television and the Aggressive Child: A Cross-National Comparison*, Lawrence Erlbaum Associates, Hillsdale, NJ.

Jago, R., Baranowski, T., Baranowski, J.C., Thompson D., Greaves K.A. (2005 June) 'BMI from 3–6 years of age is predicted by TV viewing and physical activity, not diet,' *Int J Obes*, (Lond) 29 (6): pp.557–64.

Kaiser Family Foundation (2003) *Zero to Six: Media Use in the Lives of Infants, Toddlers, and Preschoolers,* Kaiser Family Foundation, Menlo Park, CA.

Kaiser Family Foundation (2005) *Generation M: Media in the Lives of 8–18 Year Olds,* Kaiser Family Foundation, Menlo Park, CA.

Kalivas P.W., Volkow N.D. (2005) 'The neural basis of addiction: a pathology of motivation and choice,' *American Journal of Psychiatry,* 162 (8): pp.1403–13.

Kaplan & Sadock, *eds.* (1998) *Synopsis of Psychiatry,* eighth edition, Lippencott, Williams & Wilkins Baltimore, Maryland USA.

Kerwin, M.L.E. (1999) 'Empirically supported treatments in pediatric psychology: Severe feeding problems,' *Journal of Pediatric Psychology,* 24 (3), pp.193–214.

Kilpatrick, D.G., Edmunds, C. N., Seymour, A. K. (1992) *Rape in America: A report to the nation,* Arlington, TX: National Victim Center and Medical University of South Carolina.

Klesges, R.C., Shelton, M.L., Klesges, L.M. (1993 Feb) 'Effects of television on metabolic rate: potential implications for childhood obesity,' *Pediatrics,* 91(2):281-6.

Klump, K.L., Miller, K.B., Keel, P.K., McGue, M., Iacono, W.G. (May 2001) 'Genetic and environmental influences on anorexia nervosa syndromes in a population-based twin sample,' *Psychological Medicine,* 31 (4): pp.737–40.

Knight, C.A., Knight, I., Mitchell, D.C., *et al.* (2004) 'Beverage caffeine intake in US consumers and subpopulations of interest: estimates from the Share of Intake Panel survey,' *Food and Chemical Toxicology,* 42, 1923–1930.

Kortegaard, L.S., Hoerder, K., Joergensen, J, Gillberg, C., Kyvik, K.O. (Feb 2001) 'A preliminary population-based twin study of self-reported eating disorder,' *Psychological Medicine,* 31 (2): pp.361–65.

Kowalski, R.M., Limber, S.P., Agatston, P.W. (2008) *Cyber Bullying: Bullying in the Digital Age,* Blackwell, Oxford.

Large, M. (29 Sept 2006) 'Toxic TV: How the TV Medium affects children's learning': Martinhclarge@gmail.com.

Lauer, Hans E. (1981) *Aggression and Repression,* Rudolf Steiner Press, London.

Lievegoed, B. (1985) *Phases of Childhood,* Floris Books, Edinburgh.

Livingstone Black, Rosemary (2010-10-19) 'Boozy energy drink Four Loko – aka 'Blackout in a Can' – banned from N.J. college,' *Daily News* (New York).

Lobstein, T., Baur, L., Uauy, R. (2004) 'Obesity in children and young people: a crisis in public health,' *Obes Rev,* 5, supplement 1: pp.4–85.

Loh, C., Gidycz, C.A., Lobo, T.R., Luthra, R. (2005) 'A prospective analysis of sexual assault perpetration: Risk factors related to perpetrator characteristics,' *Journal of Interpersonal Violence,* 20, pp.1325–48.

Long, J.C., Knowler, W.C., Hanson, R.L. *et al.* (1998) 'Evidence for genetic linkage to alcohol dependence on chromosomes 4 and 11 from an autosome-wide scan in an American Indian population,' *American Journal of Medical Genetics. Part B: Neuropsychiatric Genetics,* 81: pp.216–21

Louw, D.A., Van Ede, D.M., Loue, A.E (1998) *Human Development* (second ed.), Kagiso Publishers, Pretoria.

Lumeng, J.C., Rahnama, S., Appugliese, D., Kaciroti, N., Bradley, R.H. (2006 April) 'Television exposure and overweight risk in preschoolers,' *Arch Pediatr Adolesc Med,* 160 (4): pp.417–22.

Martin, James A. (2000-06-09) 'The Pain of Portable Computing,' *PC World,* retrieved 2008-11-27.

Maslow, A.H. (1943) 'A Theory of Human Motivation,' *Psychological Review,* 50 (4): pp.370–96.

—, (1954) *Motivation and Personality,* Harper, New York, p.236.

Mauras, N., Rogol, A.D., Haymond, M.W., & Veldhuis, J.D. (1996) 'Sex steroids, growth hormone, insulin-like growth factor-1: Neuroendocrine and metabolic regulation in puberty,' *Hormone Research,* 45:74–80.

McCauley, K.T. *Is Addiction a Disease?* www.instituteforaddictionstudy. com.

McDonough, P. (October 26, 2009) *TV viewing among kids at an eight-year high:* http://blog.nielsen.com/nielsenwire/media.

McVey-Nobel, M., Khenlani-Patel, S., Neziroglu, F. (2006) *When your child is cutting. A parent's guide to helping children overcome self-injury,* New Harbinger Publications, Oakland CA.

Mendel, Felix (1997) 'Inclusion or delusion: can one size fit all? Educating students with special needs,' *Support for Study,* no.14, pp.152–57.

—, Atkinson, M. & Howard, J. (1997) *Controversial Issues in Special Education,* David Flanders Publishers, London.

Meier, E. (2002) 'Child Rape in South Africa,' *Pediatric Nursing,* 28 (5).

Miller, D. (2009) 'College drinking problems, deaths on the rise,' *Journal of Studies on Alcohol and Drugs,* June15 issue.

Miller, N.S., Giannini, A.J. (1990) 'The disease model of addiction: a biopsychiatrist's view,' *J. Psychoactive Drugs,* 22.

Miller, N.S., Mahler, J.C., Gold, M.S. (1991) 'Suicide risk associated

277

with drug and alcohol dependence,' *Journal of Addictive Diseases,* 10 (3): pp.49–61.

Mok, T.A. (1998) 'Getting the message: media images and stereotypes and their effect on Asian Americans,' *Cult Divers Ment Health,* 4 (3): pp.185–202.

Mooney, L. (Oct 8, 2009) *Computer Vision Syndrome:* http://www.livestrong.com/article/25560-computer-vision-syndrome/#ixzz1a5a0fIts.

Mukai, T. *et al.* (1994) 'Eating attitudes and weight preoccupation among female high school students in Japan,' *J Child Psychol Psychiatry,* 35: pp.677–88S.

Murdoch, D., Pihl, R.O., Ross, D. (1990) 'Alcohol and crimes of violence: Present issues,' *Int J Addict,* 25: 1065-81.

National Health Service (NHS) UK (2011) *Statistics on obesity, England,* Information Centre for Health and Social Care: www.ic.nhs.ukww.

Noel, J. (July 2003) 'Effects of Media on Early Brain Development,' research Paper, *Electronic Media.*

Ogden, C.L., Carroll, M.D., Flegal, K.M. (May 2008) 'High body mass index for age among US children and adolescents,' *JAMA* 299 (20): pp.2401–5: doi:10.1001/jama.299.20.2401, PMID 18505949.

Omar, S., Wild, A. (2005) *Research into the Dynamics of Young Sex Offenders in Venda,* Research conducted for Thouyandou Victim Empowerment Trust.

Outram, S.M. (2010) 'The use of methylphenidate among students: the future of enhancement?' *J. Med. Ethics,* 36(4): pp.198-20.

Palmer, Shirley (1984) 'Transient Myopia after Visual Work,' *Ergonomics,* Vol.2, No.11.

—, (1993) 'Does computer use put children's vision at risk?' *Journal of Research and Development in Education,* Vol.26, No.2, pp.59–65.

Palmer, Sue (2007) *Toxic Childhood,* Orion Books, London.

Parliamentary Office of Science and Technology (July 2005) *Binge Drinking and Public Health,* Number 244.

Parry, C., Morojele, N., Jernigan, D. (2002) *Action for a Sober South Africa,* Alcohol & Drug Abuse Research Unit, South African Medical Research Council.

Pascarelli, E., Quilter, D. (1994) *Repetitive Strain Injury: A Computer User's Guide,* Wiley Publishers, NY.

Patzlaff, R. (1988) *Medienmagie und die Herrschaft ueber die Sinne (Magic of the Media, Tyranny over the Senses),* Verlag Freies Geistesleben, Stuttgart.

Pelkonen, M., Martunen, M. (2003) 'Child and adolescent suicide: epidemiology, risk factors, and approaches to prevention,' *Paediat Drugs,*5 (4): pp.243–65.

Pich, E.M., Pagliusi, S.R.,Tessari, M., Talabot-Ayer, D., Hooft Van Huijsduijnen, R., Chiamulera, C. (1997) 'Common neural substrates for the addictive properties of nicotine and cocaine,' *Science* 275 (5296): pp.83–86.

Pike, K.M., Rodin, J. (1991) 'Mothers, daughters and disordered eating,' *Journal of Abnormal Psychology,* 97: pp.198–204.

Pollak, C.P. & Bright, D. (2003) 'Caffeine consumption and weekly sleep patterns in US seventh-, eighth-, and ninth-graders,' *Pediatrics,* 111, pp.42–46.

Postman, N. (1986) *Amusing Ourselves to Death,* Heinemann, London.

—, (1993) *Technopoly The Surrender of Culture to Technology,* Vintage Books, New York.

—, (1994) *The Disappearance of Childhood,* Vintage Books, New York.

Rang, Dale & Ritter *eds,* (1995) *Pharmacology,* third edition, Churchill Livingstone, UK.

Rayworth, B.B., Wise, L.A., Harlow, B.H. (2004) 'Child Abuse and Risk of Eating Disorders in Women,' *Epidemiology,* Volume 15, No.3, pp.271–78.

Rehm, J. *et al.* (2003) 'Alcohol-related morbidity and mortality,' *Alcohol Research and Health,* 27 (1): pp.39-51.

Reich, T., Edenberg, H.J., Goate, A. *et al.* (1998) 'Genome-wide search for genes affecting the risk for alcohol dependence,' *American Journal of Medical Genetics,* 81: pp.207–215.

Rideout, V.J., Foehr, U.G., Roberts, D.F. (January 2010) *Media in the lives of 8-18* Gigli, S., (April 2004) *Children,Youth and Media Around the World: An Overview of Trends & Issues,* Inter Media Survey Institute, for UNICEF.

Rideout, V.J., Vandewater, E.A., Wartella, E.A. (2003) *Zero to six: electronic media in the lives of infants, toddlers and preschoolers,* Kaiser Family Foundation, Menlo Park CA.

Robin, A.L., Gilroy, M., Dennis, A.B. (1998) 'Treatment of Eating Disorders in Children and Adolescents,' *Clinical Psychology Review,* 18 (4): pp.421–46.

Rosemary, T. (2006) *Most at risk are young males between 17 and 25 years,* Royal Society for the Prevention of Accidents Conference Proceedings.

Russell, M. (1990) 'Prevalence of alcoholism among children of alcoholics.' In: Windle, M., Searles, J.S., *eds. Children of Alcoholics: Critical Perspectives,* Guilford, New York, pp.9–38.

Sachsse, U., Von Der Heyde, S., G. Huether (2002) 'Stress regulation and self-mutilation,' *Americal Journal of Psychiatry,* 159(4): p.672.

Sanders, B. (1994) *A is for Ox: Violence, Electronic Media and the Silencing of the Written Word,* Pantheon, NY.

Schewe, P.A. (2006) *Interventions to prevent sexual violence.* In L.S. Doll, S.E. Bonzo, J.A. Mercy, D.A. Sleet, eds. *Handbook of Injury and Violence Prevention,* pp.223–40, Springer, NY.

Searle, J.R. (1992) *The Rediscovery of the Mind,* MIT Press, USA.

Senate Judiciary Committee Media Violence Report (1999) *Children, Violence and the Media.*

Serdula, M.K., Ivery, D., Coates, R.J., Freedman, D.S., Williamson, D.F., Byers, T. (2002) *Do Obese Children Become Obese Adults? A Review of the Literature,* National Center for Chronic Disease Prevention, Atlanta, USA.

Shaw, D., Fernandes, J.R., Chitra, R., (December 2005) 'Suicide in Children and Adolescents: A 10-Year Retrospective Review,' *American Journal of Forensic Medicine & Pathology,* Vol.26, 4, pp.309–315.

Shaw, J. (2000) 'Child on child sexual abuse: Psychological perspectives,' *Child Abuse & Neglect,* 24 (12): pp.1591–1600.

Sloan, D. (1985) *The Computer in Education: A Critical perspective,* Teachers College Press, NY.

Smith, G.T., Goldman, M.S., Greenbaum, P.E., Christiansen, B.A. (1995) 'Expectancy for social facilitation from drinking: The divergent paths of high-expectancy and low-expectancy adolescents,' *Journal of Abnormal Psychology,* 104: pp.32–40.

Spear, L.P. (2000) 'The adolescent brain and age-related behavioral manifestations,' *Neuroscience and Biobehavioral Reviews,* 24: pp.417–63.

—, & Varlinskaya, E.I. (2005) 'Adolescence: Alcohol sensitivity, tolerance, and intake.' In: Galanter, M., ed. *Recent Developments in Alcoholism,* Vol. 17: *Alcohol Problems in Adolescents and Young Adults: Epidemiology, Neurobiology, Prevention, Treatment,* Springer, NY, pp.143–59.

Stanton, W. (1992) 'A longitudinal study of the influence of parents and friends on children's initiation of smoking,' *Journal of Applied Developmental Psychology,* 13 (4): pp.423–34.

Steele, R. (2005) 'A hermeneutic phenomenological study of/in transformation: An embodied and creative exploration of therapeutic change through Psychophonetics psychotherapy.' Doctoral thesis. Edith Cowan University, Western Australia.

—, (2011) *Psychophonetics: Holistic Counseling and Psychotherapy: Stories and Insights from Practice,* Lindisfarne Books, NY.

Steinberger, J., Moran, A., Hong, C.P., Jacobs, D.R. Jr, Sinaiko, A.R. (2001) 'Adiposity in childhood predicts obesity and insulin resistance in young adulthood,' *J Pediatr,* 138: pp.469–73.

Steiner, Rudolf (1904/1971) *Theosophy: an introduction to the super-sensible knowledge of the world and the destination of the human being,* Anthroposophic Press, New York.

—, (1908/1973) *Lectures on The Gospel of St John,* May 23, Anthroposophic Press, Spring Valley, NY.

—, (1910/1999) *A Psychology of Body, Soul and Spirit,* four lectures, Nov 1–4, 1910, Anthroposophic Press, Hudson, NY.

—, (1910/1997) *An Outline of Esoteric Science,* Anthroposophic Press, Hudson, NY.

—, (1918) 'The Work of the Angels in Man's Astral Body,' October 9 lecture in Zurich.

—, (1921/1978) 'Knowledge of Man and the Form of the Lesson,' June 13 lecture, Bibliography (GA) 302, Rudolf Steiner Press.

—, (1921/1981) *Study of Man,* Rudolf Steiner Press, London.

—, (1922/1976) *Lectures to the Workmen in Dornach,* Steiner Verlag, Dornach, Switzerland.

—, (1975) *Education of the Child,* Rudolf Steiner Press, London.

Stolle, M., Sack, P.M., Thomasius, R. (May 2009) 'Binge drinking in childhood and adolescence: epidemiology, consequences, and interventions,' *Dtsch Arztebl Int,* 106 (19): pp.323–28.

Strauss, R.S., Barlow, S.E., Dietz, W.H. (2000) 'Prevalence of abnormal serum aminotransferase values in overweight and obese adolescents,' *Journal of Pediatrics,* 136: pp.727–33.

Szabo, C.P. (1997) 'Abnormal Eating Attitudes in Secondary School Girls in South Africa – a preliminary study,' *SA Med J,* 4, supplement, pp.524-26, 528-30.

—, (April 1997) 'Factors influencing eating attitudes in secondary-school girls in South Africa – a preliminary study,' *South African Med J,* Vol. 87, No.4.

Tagar, Y., Goldberg, R, 'Transforming the Enemy: A Psycho-spiritual-somatic Approach to Auto-Immune Disorders using Medical Psychophonetics. A Foundation Paper for Participatory Medicine.' (Unpublished article)

Tagar, Y. (1986–2006) *Psychophonetics: A Collection of Articles,* IAPP: www.psychophonetics.co..au /pages/articles.html.

Tamburro, R.F., Gordon, P.L, D'Apolito, J.P., Howard, S.C. (2004 Dec) 'Unsafe and violent behavior in commercials aired during televised major sporting events,' *Pediatrics,* 114 (6): pp.694–98.

Tapert, S.F., Schweinsburg, A.D. (2005) 'The human adolescent brain and alcohol use disorders.' In: Galanter, M., ed. *Recent Developments in Alcoholism,* Vol. 17: *Alcohol Problems in Adolescents and Young*

Adults: Epidemiology, Neurobiology, Prevention, Treatment, Springer, NY, pp.177–97.

Thakkar, R.R., Garrison, M.M., Christakis, D.A. (2006) 'A systematic review for the effects of television viewing by infants and preschoolers,' *Pediatrics,* 118: pp.2025–2031.

Valdemar,W., Setzer, V.W., Duckett, G.E. (1992) *The Risks to Children using Electronic Games,* Proceedings Vol. 2, p.471.

Valek, M., Laslavic, B. & Laslavic, Z. (2004) 'Daily caffeine intake among Osijek High School students: questionnaire study,' *Croatian Medical Journal,* 45, pp.72–75.

Viner, R.M., Cole, T.J. (2005) 'Television viewing in early childhood predicts adult body mass index,' *J Pediatr,* Oct. 147 (4): pp.429–35.

Vitale, S., Sperduto, R.D., Ferris, F.L., (December 2009) *Increased prevalence of myopia in the United States between 1971-1972 and 1999-2004,* Archives of Ophthalmology.

Vogt, F. (2002) *Addiction's Many Faces,* Hawthorn Press, Stroud, UK.

Walters, P.A., (March 2010) 'Promiscuity in Adolescence,' *American Journal of Orthopsychiatry.*

Wang, Y., Lobstein, T. (2006) 'Worldwide trends in childhood overweight and obesity.' *International Journal of Pediatric Obesity,* Vol.1, No.1, pp.11–25.

Welsh, J.A., Sharma, A., Cunningham, S.A., Vos, M.B. (2011) 'Consumption of Added Sugars and Indicators of Cardiovascular Disease Risk among US Adolescents,' *Circulation,* 123: pp.249–57.

White, R. (2006) *How Computers Work,* eighth edition, Que Publishing, Indianapolis.

Williams, C.L. *et al.* (2002) 'Cardiovascular Health in Childhood,' *Circulation,* 106: pp.143–160.

Willis, B.M., Levy, B.S., (2002) 'Child prostitution: global health burden, research needs, and interventions,' *The Lancet,* V359 (9315), pp.1417–22.

Winchel, R., Stanley, M. (1991) 'Self-injurious behaviour: A review of the behaviour and biology of self-mutilation,' *American Journal of Psychiatry,* 148: pp.306–17.

Wolak, J., Mitchell K.J., Finkelhor, D. (2007) 'Does online harassment constitute bullying? An exploration of online harassment by known peers and online-only contacts,' *Journal of Adolescent Health,* 41 (supplement 1): pp.S51–58.

Wood, P.B. (2008) 'Role of central dopamine in pain and analgesia,' *Expert Rev Neurother,* 8 (5): pp.781–97.

World Health Organization (2001) *World Report on Violence and Health,* Geneva, Switzerland.

—, (2002) *World Report on Violence and Health. Drugs, Alcohol and Violence,* Geneva, Switzerland.

World Health Organization Global Status (2004) *Report on Alcohol,* Geneva, Switzerland.

Wyclif, William (1989) *The Harmony of Birds,* Floris Books, Edinburgh.

Zimmerman, F.J., Christakis, D.A. (2005) 'Children's television viewing and cognitive outcomes: a longitudinal analysis of national data,' *Arch Pediatr Adolesc Med,* July, 159 (7): pp.619–25.

Index